Praise for Please Don't Eat the Animals

"A pocket battleship of ammunition to use in debating those who consider meat-eating an inalienable right."

—Chris Mercer and Beverley Pervan, *Animal People*

"As easy to read as it is to say "veggie burger." In a few words, this book gives you one good reason after the other to follow a good diet, from reducing high blood pressure to conserving top soil, from livening up your menu and your life to being able to look a cow in the eye without feeling guilty."

—Ingrid E. Newkirk, president,
People for the Ethical Treatment of Animals (PETA)

"I can remember when someone who ate food that was unhealthy, that was produced in a way that did serious damage to the environment and caused immense suffering to animals, was considered normal. While someone who ate food that was healthy, and produced in an Earth-friendly way without any cruelty was considered a health nut. But all that is changing. If you read this book, you will be far more able to make your food choices align with your values. And your body will thank you for the rest of your life."

—John Robbins, *Healthy at 100, Diet for a New America*, and *The Food Revolution*

"This exciting and easy-to-read book succinctly presents the key reasons to stop eating animals. As you will see, vegetarians enjoy healthier and longer lives while preserving the earth's precious resources. Most importantly, we go to sleep at night knowing that our choices have greatly reduced suffering in the world."

—Stewart David, president, Carolina Animal Action

continued...

“...a reference for those of us who shun meat, and a handbook for our friends who are still on the fence.”

—Joseph Connelly, founder and publisher, *VegNews Magazine*

“Bravo to the authors for presenting a concise and easy-to-comprehend case for why adopting a vegetarian lifestyle is the road map to a better world for all. This book should be circulated in libraries and schools. I wholeheartedly recommend it.”

—Eric Brent, founder, HappyCow's Vegetarian Guide to Restaurants and Health Food Stores (www.happycow.net)

Please Don't Eat the Animals

All the Reasons You Need to Be a Vegetarian

Jennifer Horsman & Jaime Flowers

Sanger, California

Printed in the United States of America

Published by Quill Driver Books/Word Dancer Press, Inc.
1254 Commerce Way
Sanger, California 93657
559-876-2170 • 1-800-497-4909 • FAX 559-876-2180

QuillDriverBooks.com
Info@QuillDriverBooks.com

Quill Driver Books/Word Dancer Press, Inc. project cadre:
Stewart David, Mary Ann Gardner, Doris Hall, Wendy Means,
Stephen Blake Mettee, Carlos Olivas, Andrea Wright

Quill Driver Books and colophon are trademarks of
Quill Driver Books/Word Dancer Press, Inc.
First printing

ISBN 1-884956-60-2

Library of Congress Cataloging-in-Publication Data

1. Horsman, Jennifer, 1957-
Please don't eat the animals : all the reasons you need to be a vegetarian / by Jennifer Horsman & Jaime Flowers.
p. cm.
Includes bibliographical references and index.
ISBN 1-884956-60-2
1. Vegetarianism. 2. Vegetarian cookery. 3. Meat--Health aspects.
4. Vegetarianism--Religious aspects.
I. Flowers, Jaime, 1984- II. Title.
RM236.H66 2006
613.2'62--dc22

2006029610

This book is dedicated to Dr. Peter Singer who is destined to appear in the history books as our century's greatest philosopher.

CONTENTS

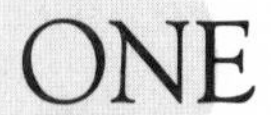

ONE

The Healthy Vegetarian

"Nothing will benefit human health and increase chances for survival of life on earth as much as the evolution to a vegetarian diet."

—Albert Einstein

Health and vegetarianism go together. If this is in any way a surprise, you haven't been paying attention to the preponderance of nutritional and medical research that advocates plant-based diets for everyone. Meat-based diets are weighted with unhealthy fats, too much protein, and loaded with calories, pesticides, hormones, and other chemicals. Meat might be what's for dinner, but it definitely is not what's good for our health.

In dramatic contrast, healthy vegetarian diets are full of fruits and vegetables, plenty of fiber, tons of nutrients, less saturated fats, and less cholesterol.

Additionally, plant-based diets are comprised of a far greater variety of foods, making these diets not just more healthful and nutritious but also more exciting and fun.

Hundreds upon hundreds of scientific articles from around the world demonstrate that a healthy vegetarian diet is the single most powerful thing individuals can do to promote, protect, or improve their health.

"Each year, the meat industrial complex abuses and butchers nearly 9 billion cows, pigs, sheep, turkeys, chickens, and other innocent, feeling animals just for the enjoyment of consumers. Each year, nearly 1.5 million of these consumers are crippled and killed prematurely by heart failure, cancer, stroke, and other chronic diseases that have been linked conclusively with the consumption of these animals. Each year, millions of other animals are abused and sacrificed in a vain search for a 'magic pill' that would vanquish these largely self-inflicted diseases."

—Alex Hershaft, Ph.D., president, Farm Animal Reform Movement

Types of Vegetarians

Vegetarian: A person who doesn't eat meat, fish or fowl.

Lacto-Ovo Vegetarian: A person who doesn't eat meat, fish, or fowl, but does eat eggs and dairy products.

Ovo-Vegetarian: A person who doesn't eat meat, fish, fowl, or dairy products, but does eat eggs.

Lacto-Vegetarian: A person who doesn't eat meat, fish, fowl, or eggs, but does eat dairy products.

Vegan: A person who doesn't eat meat, fish, fowl, eggs, or any dairy products. Most vegans also do not use any animal products such as leather or fur either.

> "*The animals of the world exist for their own reasons. They were not made for humans any more than black people were made for whites or women for men.*"
>
> —Alice Walker, author, *The Color Purple*

> *"Certainly, a sort of industrial use of creatures, so that geese are fed in such a way as to produce as large a liver as possible, or hens live so packed together that they become just caricatures of birds, this degrading of living creatures to a commodity seems to me in fact to contradict the relationship of mutuality that comes across in the Bible."*
>
> —Pope Benedict XVI

Strong and Healthy Hearts

Heart disease is the leading cause of death and disability in the world; according to the World Health Federation it kills almost 17 million people a year, stealing more lives prematurely than all other causes of death combined. A stunning 41.6 percent of all deaths in the United States last year were caused by cardiovascular diseases. Worldwide, more women die from heart disease than the next seven most common causes of death. A plethora of large-scale scientific studies shows that a plant-based diet prevents deaths from heart attacks:

- When analyzing 8,300 deaths in the United States, United Kingdom, and Germany among 76,000 men and women in five different, large studies, researchers concluded that vegetarians have a 24 percent reduction in death from heart disease (Key et al., 1998).

- Similarly, in the famous Oxford Vegetarian Study where 6,000 vegetarians were compared with 5,000 meat eaters over nearly two decades, scientists found that the rate of death from heart disease was 28 percent lower in vegetarians than in meat eaters (Thorogood et al., 1994).

- Furthermore, vegans, men and women who eat no meat, dairy products, or eggs, have a whopping 57 percent lower incidence of death from heart disease (Thorogood et al., 1990).

- Do healthy meat eaters—people who don't smoke, who exercise a lot, and consume a low-fat meat diet—enjoy the same heart healthy benefits provided by the vegetarian diet? Scientists compared vegetarians to healthy meat eaters, and vegetarians still had far lower rates of both heart disease and deaths from heart disease (Mann et al., 1997; Chang-Claude et al., 2005).

Jim, age 48, of Idaho, describes what happened to him:

> I never thought a moment about food. I ate it all, and a lot of it was meat; dinner wasn't dinner without meat, and lunch was often a giant sandwich with the meat piled an inch high, and milk. Running my feed store, lifting fifty-pound bags all the time, I figured I got enough exercise.

Wrong. I started feelin' a little tired—that was my only warning. One morning before my first cup of coffee, it struck. Like a 9.0 earthquake. A massive heart attack—the pain ricocheted head to toe, squeezing my chest, ripping my breath from me. I thought I was going to die; I knew I was going to die. But I got lucky and the paramedics got to me on time. The damage to my heart was not so bad, but I needed a triple bypass. For six weeks afterward, I could barely move. Lost thirty pounds. I never want to go through that again.

My doctor drew the connection between fat intake, meat, and heart disease for me, and she recommended a book by Dr. Dean Ornish—a vegetarian program to fight heart disease. My wife was all gung-ho; I think my heart attack scared her more than it scared me! She informed me that we'd literally try anything.

We've been vegetarians for two years now. At first I thought it would be real hard, but well, I guess that was the big surprise...and how much better I feel—lighter and healthier. Oh, sure, every once in a while I'll get a hankerin' for a burger, but I just think back to the months of pain and recovery, and that cravin' goes by real quick.

Heart Health: The Contributing Factors

Not only do vegetarians have lower rates of death from coronary artery disease, they have much less of the disease itself.

- One study analyzed eighty scientific studies in leading medical journals. The analysis found that vegetarians had lower blood pressure, were slimmer, and were less likely to suffer from stroke, heart attack, and kidney failure (Barnard et al., 2005).

- A large German study of nearly 2,000 vegetarians found that deaths from heart disease were reduced by over one-third, and that heart disease itself was far less than that of the general population (Chang-Claude et al., 1992).

- Still another large study examined the coronary artery disease risk of young adults ages 18 to 30, and vegetarians were found to have much higher levels of cardiovascular fitness and—once again—a greatly reduced risk of heart disease (Slatter,y et al. 1991). Additionally, diet researchers at the University of Minnesota studied teenage vegetarians, discovering that these young people ate a far healthier diet than their meat-eating peers.

"The process of gradual blocking of the coronary arteries begins not in adulthood but in childhood...and the main cause of this arteriosclerosis is the steadily increasing amount of fat in the American diet, particularly saturated animals fats such as those found in meat, chicken, milk and cheeses. If there was another disease that caused half a million deaths a year, you can be sure that the public would be acutely aware of the danger, and that the cure or prevention would be practiced universally."

—Dr. Benjamin Spock,
author, child expert

The Cholesterol Culprit

Many scientists have concluded that the major risk factor in heart disease is cholesterol. The only foods that contain cholesterol are animal products, and so vegetarians have fewer cholesterol worries. Literally hundreds of studies make the point:

- Countless studies have found, like the Oxford Vegetarian study, that vegetarians had significantly lower cholesterol levels (Thorogood et al., 1994).

- When people begin eating a plant-based diet, they reduce their blood cholesterol levels from an average high of 237mg/dL to a normal level of 137mg/dL (Anderson et al., 1995).

- It has been shown that a vegetarian diet rich in fruits, vegetables, and nuts reduces cholesterol levels better than our best medicine. (Jenkins et al. 2003b).

- Lower your cholesterol by simply reducing the amount of meat you eat, keeping in mind that a mere 10 percent reduction in blood cholesterol levels can significantly lower your chances of getting a heart attack by 30 percent. This potent effect is seen in epidemiological studies around the world. People in China and Japan consume far less meat, and their cholesterol levels are much lower than people in the big meat eating countries. (Campbell and Campbell, 2006).

"I don't understand why asking people to eat a well-balanced vegetarian diet is considered drastic, while it is medically conservative to cut people open and put them on powerful cholesterol-lowering drugs for the rest of their lives."

—Dr. Dean Ornish, author,
Reversing Heart Disease

Blood Pressure

Sometimes called the silent killer and a major risk factor for heart disease, high blood pressure affects approximately 1 billion people worldwide, but fortunately vegetarians benefit from much lower blood pressure. On average, vegetarians' systolic blood pressure (the upper number) is 9.3 percent lower than meat eaters', while their diastolic blood pressure (the lower number) is 18.2 percent lower (Lyman and Merzer, 1997).

- Over 30 percent of meat eaters suffer from high blood pressure (Mackay and Mensah, 2004), but less than 4 percent of vegetarians experience higher than normal blood pressure, and "going vegan" virtually guarantees low blood pressure.

- In a study that attempted to control for other health factors, researchers examined Trappist monks, who are vegetarians, and compared them with Benedictines, who are not. With the meat exception, both groups have remarkably similar lifestyles. The Trappist monks had much lower blood pressure (Barnard et al., 2005).

- Studies have shown that when hypertensive patients adopt a vegetarian diet, they experience a marked decrease in blood pressure. In one such study, even people with normal blood pressure who adopted a vegetarian diet, experienced a five-point drop in systolic pressure (the upper number) and a two to three point drop in diastolic pressure (Barnard et al., 2005). For many people, a vegetarian diet works better than our best blood pressure medicine and with none of the troubling side effects of such medications—like impotence.

- Black people appear to have a predisposition to high blood pressure, and the vegetarian diet works especially well in lowering this vital sign for people of color (Melby et al., 1993).

Jean Ann from Georgia tells her story about lowering blood pressure and cholesterol:

> My dad died of a heart attack when he was only 45, and my mother died of one at 63. Not being an idiot, these events scared the heck out of me: I watched my weight, exercised every day, and tried to eat right. No matter what I did though, both my blood pressure and cholesterol were off-the-charts high. My doctor kept trying different medicines on me. We finally found one that lowered my blood pressure into a high-normal range without too many side effects, but none of the medicines managed to lower my cholesterol. It stayed "damn high," as my doctor said. He finally suggested I give up meat, which, I might add, is no easy feat in the south. It was kind of hard at first, but after just two months my blood pressure fell to low-normal, and my cholesterol dropped into a normal range! Here's the really weird part—somehow over the course of those first two months I lost my taste for meat, any and all kinds of it. I don't think I'll ever eat it again.

The more you go vegetarian, the healthier your heart will be. On a spectrum with daily meat eating at one end, vegetarianism in the middle and veganism at the other end, the closer we move toward vegan, the less cardiovascular disease we have (Thorogood et al,. 1994).

> "*...Meat can never be a healthy food: it is pain-poisoned.*"
>
> —Sri Swami Satchidananda, founder Intregral Yoga, and author, *The Healthy Vegetarian*

Let's Not Forget Strokes

Across North America and Europe, stroke is the third leading cause of death behind heart disease and cancer. Stroke is also the most common cause of long-term disability among adults in the United States. Vegetarians have a 20 to 30 percent reduced risk of having a stroke; vegans have a hugely reduced risk of ever having a stroke. Stroke, like heart disease, is associated with diets high in saturated fats (Sasaki et al., 1995) and the vegetarian diet is naturally low in these fats.

> "*The Gods created certain kinds of beings to replenish our bodies... they are the trees and the plants and the seeds....*"
>
> —Plato

Cancer

Vegetarians have far lower rates of cancer. More than 10 million people worldwide are diagnosed with cancer each year, and unfortunately this number is rising; it is estimated that there will be 15 million new cases per year by 2020. Cancer causes 6.7 million deaths every year—or 12 percent of deaths worldwide. In addition to the enormous personal costs of these deadly diseases, cancer is one of the most expensive medical conditions: For instance, in the United States alone almost 1.4 million people are annually diagnosed with cancer at a cost of about $77.1 billion a year, according to the National Cancer Institute.

Going vegetarian protects people against many, if not most, cancers, as scientists estimate that between 40 and 70 percent of cancer mortality is related to diet. As with heart disease, no one knows for certain whether the protection offered by a vegetarian diet is the result of the increased vegetables or the absence of meat, but lately the evidence is coming down on the side of the absence of meat.

In other words, while vegetables are an important part of a healthy diet and plant foods contain myriad nutrients, and many of these are potent anti-carcinogens, it appears that meat consumption and cancer go together. Some larger international studies on vegetarians and cancer rates support this:

- The Oxford Vegetarian Study found cancer

mortality to be 39 percent lower among vegetarians when compared to with meat-eaters (Appleby et al., 1999).

- A long-term, ongoing study that began in the 1960s of the largely vegetarian Seventh Day Adventists conducted by Loma Linda University has found cancer mortality rates to be much lower than those of the general population for several cancer sites unrelated to smoking or alcohol consumption.

- The European Prospective Investigation of Cancer found that vegetarians suffer 40 percent fewer cancers than the general population.

- Based on hundreds of international dietary studies, the World Cancer Research Fund's and the World Health Organization's dietary advice urge people to reduce the intake of dietary fat and increase the consumption of fruits, vegetables and whole grains, or in other words—go vegetarian.

"Insecticides, fecal contamination, pesticides, products used in paint and preservation of wood, hormones, and animal drugs all turn up in meat."

—Carol Tucker Foreman, former Assistant U.S. Secretary of Agriculture

Join the Crowd

By becoming a vegetarian, you join a select group of the world's greatest thinkers, scientists, philosophers, artists and writers, and a bunch of Hollywood folks. The extensive list of famous vegetarian philosophers, scientists, and Nobel Prize winners includes:

> Confucius, Buddha, Hesiod, Pythagoras, Socrates, Plato, Diogenes, Epicurus, Ovid, Seneca, Plutarch, Plotinus, Porphyry, Iamblichus, Leonardo da Vinci, Voltaire, Oliver Goldsmith, Jean-Jacques Rousseau, Benjamin Franklin, Thomas Jefferson, Newton, Charles Darwin, Jeremy Bentham, Arthur Schopenhauer, Susan B. Anthony, Thomas Edison, Dr. Albert Schweitzer, Albert Einstein, Gandhi, Norman Cousins, Dr. Benjamin Spock, Jane Goodall, Tom Regan, and Dr. Peter Singer.

Famous vegetarian writers and artists include:

> Scott Adams, Louisa May Alcott, Clive Barker, Berkeley Breathed, Charlotte Bronte, Lord Byron, J. M. Coetzee, Alberto Chavez, Ted Hughs, Arianna Huffington, Franz Kafka, Frances Moore Lappe, Hans Christian Anderson, V. S. Naipaul, John Robbins, Anthony Robbins, Henry Salt, George Bernard Shaw, Mary Wollstonecraft Shelley, Percy Bysshe Shelley, Isaac Bashevis Singer, Leo Tolstoy, Thomas Tyron, Alice Walker, and Margaret Atwood.

Many Hollywood folks have gone vegetarian, and these smart celebrities include:

Casey Affleck, Gillian Anderson, Pamela Anderson, Bea Arthur, Bill Maher, Alec Baldwin, Brigitte Bardot, Drew Barrymore, Kim Basinger, Meredith Baxter, Orlando Bloom, Peter Bogdanovich, Ellen Burstyn, John Cleese, George Clooney, James Cromwell, Ted Danson, Danny DeVito, Cameron Diaz, Leonardo DiCaprio, David Duchovny, Michael J. Fox, Janeane Garofalo, Richard Gere, Sir John Gielgud, Valerie Harper, Woody Harrelson, Josh Hartnett, Dustin Hoffman, Katie Holmes, Jude Law, Cloris Leachman, Julia Louis-Dreyfus, Madonna, Tobey Maguire, Sir Ian McKellen, Hayley Mills, Demi Moore, Esai Morales, Brittany Murphy, Paul Newman, Gwyneth Paltrow, Anna Paquin, Guy Pearce, Joaquin Phoenix, Rain Phoenix, Brad Pitt, Natalie Portman, Stephanie Powers, Robin Raven, Joe Regalbuto, Julia Roberts, Steven Seagal, Martin Shaw, Brooke Shields, Alicia Silverstone, Paul McCartney, Julia Stiles, Eric Stoltz, Peter Sumner, Liv Tyler, Mary Tyler-Moore, Vince Vaughn, Lindsay Wagner, Naomi Watts, Dennis Weaver, Kate Winslet, Reese Witherspoon, and Lisa Simpson.

Breast Cancer

Vegetarians have lower rates of breast cancer. Worldwide, more than a million women are diagnosed with breast cancer every year, which accounts for 23 percent of all women's cancer cases. Incidence rates vary considerably, but the highest rates of breast cancer occur in countries that consume the most meat, and this is no coincidence. To prevent breast cancer or to stop its devastating effects, going vegetarian provides a meaningful measure of protection:

- A meta-analysis of studies on dietary fat and breast cancer found that a strong correlation exists between the two (Boyd, 1993).

- The British Department of Health conducted a large-scale analysis of ten cohort studies on breast cancer and dietary factors and found an elevated risk for breast cancer in meat eaters. The more meat one consumes, the greater the risk; women who ate meat every day were at the highest risk (Bingham & Wilcock, 1999).

- Scientists at the Cornell University Program of Breast Cancer and Environmental Risk Factors examined fifteen recent studies of meat consumption and breast cancer, twelve of which demonstrated that meat consumption affects the risk of contracting breast cancer. Indeed the association between meat consumption and breast cancer risk was dramatic in many of these studies. Like the previous analysis, a number of these studies showed that the quantity of meat consumed affects breast cancer risk, with the less meat a woman eats, the lower her risk of ever contracting this disease.

- Studies have also shown that decreasing a woman's animal fat intake can reduce the chances that she will die from the disease. This is an amazing fact that definitely deserves more publicity (Zhang et al., 1995).

Nancy, 48, of California relates:

> I'm an identical twin, or I was until my sister, Karen, died of breast cancer. The only difference between us? I've been a vegetarian since my teens and weighed about ten pounds less. I'm not saying this is proof that being a vegetarian shields you from cancer, 'cause we're only two people, and obviously everyone is different. But if there is any chance that it helps you, for heaven's sake, go for it. You'll get some cancer protection, a healthier heart, you won't be hurting any animals, and you'll be doing something good for the environment.

Prostate Cancer

Prostate cancer is the most common form of cancer other than skin cancers and the second leading cause of cancer deaths among men in the United States, Europe, and throughout much of the rest of the world. It is estimated that 70 percent of men who reach age 80 will have the disease. And, as with so many other cancers, a vegetarian diet plays a definitive role in prevention and, even treatment.

- A large-scale, long-term study in the Netherlands found a powerful connection between the amount of animal fats consumed and the rate of prostate cancer (Schuurman et al., 1999).

- A review of a dozen studies found dietary fat strongly correlated with prostate cancer (Giovannucci et al., 1993).

- Other scientists conducted a thorough review of the scientific research on risk factors involved in prostate cancer and reached the same conclusion: The less fat from meat that a man consumes, the lower his chances of getting prostate cancer. (Pienta & Esper, 1993).

- Most studies have found that the more fruits and vegetables a man consumes, the less chance of his getting prostate cancer (Cohen et al., 2000).

- Studies have also shown that once a man is diagnosed with prostate cancer, his survival rate increases if he goes vegetarian, and that even a reduction of animal fats will increase his survival rate (Meyer et al., 1999).

Intestinal Cancers

Similarly, international studies have measured the consumption of animal fats and rates of intestinal cancers, and these all have found that the more animal fat consumed, the higher the rate of these devastating diseases. The latest research found that meat eating increases your chance of contracting colon cancer by a whopping 50 percent (Chao et al., 2005).

Gary of New Mexico tells this cautionary tale:

> My mom died of colon cancer. By the time they caught it, it was too late. I stayed with her 24/7 in the end… All I can say is no one on earth deserves that much pain. No one. If being a vegetarian offers any chance of reducing the odds of contracting this disease, my God, sign me up. Sign up everyone.

Other Cancers

> *"How good it is to be well fed, healthy, and kind all at the same time."*
>
> —Dr. Henry Heimlich, inventor of the Heimlich Maneuver

Dr. Dean Edell, the popular radio physician, reports that a vegetarian smoker has less chance of getting lung cancer than a nonsmoking meat eater. Even controlling for smoking, vegetarians have much lower rates of lung cancer (Deneco-Pellegrini et al., 1996).

> *"In my view, no chemical carcinogen is nearly so important in causing human cancer as animal protein."*
>
> —Dr. T. Colin Campbell,
> author, *The China Health Study*

Ovarian, uterine, and endometrial cancers have all been shown to be strongly correlated to the amount of animal fat in one's diet, and vegetarian women have significantly lower rates of these cancers (Risch et al., 1994).

> *"The beef industry has contributed to more American deaths than all the wars of this century, all the natural disasters, and all automobile accidents combined."*
>
> — Dr. Neal Barnard, director of
> Physicians for Responsible
> Medicine

Vegetarians have much stronger immune systems (Malter et al., 1989), and many scientists theorize that this fact contributes to the amazingly lower cancer rates found in vegetarians.

Killer Diabetes

Vegetarians have *far* lower rates of type 2 diabetes and are far less likely to die of diabetes and its related risk factors than meat eaters. (Brathwaite et al., 2003). The latest World Health Organization estimate for the number of people with diabetes worldwide is 177 million. This figure is likely to more than double by 2030. Overall, direct health-care costs of diabetes range from 2.5 percent to 15 percent of annual health-care budgets, depending on the prevalence of diabetes and the sophistication of the treatment available. A lifelong disease that can be dangerous, diabetes has become a golbal epidemic. Eventually it causes damage to the nerves and blood vessels, leaving individuals at increased risk for eye, heart, blood vessel, nerve, and kidney disease. It is strongly linked to meat-loaded diets high in saturated fat and shares all the common markers of coronary heart disease: raised cholesterol levels, elevated blood pressure, and obesity.

Tragically, this disease now appears in our children as well. Appearing with skyrocketing rates of childhood obesity, type 2 diabetes is becoming increasingly common throughout North America, Europe, and even some Asian countries such as Japan and Thailand. Once an individual is diagnosed, the current dietary prescription is a regimen high in carbohydrates, high in fiber, and low in fat—in other words, a vegetarian diet. Indeed, studies have shown that the vegetarian diet can be a *cure* for many type 2 diabetics (Jenkins et al. 2003b).

The Growing Problem—Obesity

Vegetarians have lower rates of obesity than meat eaters; the body mass index of vegetarians is closer to the desired 20-25 BMI than that of the rest of the population (Pi-Snyder, 1991). This is seen throughout the world. Following the same dynamics as diabetes, weight problems and obesity have become a worldwide epidemic: More than 1 billion adults are overweight, and at least 300 million of them are clinically obese. The United States amplifies these statistics: 127 million Americans are overweight, 60 million are obese, and 9 million are severely obese. While these rates are rising substantially throughout all of North and South America and Europe, obesity has now emerged even in traditionally slender populations such as China and Japan.

This epidemic has reached our young people as well: 15.5 percent of adolescents and 15.3 percent of children are obese in North America, an alarming increase in recent years. These figures for childhood obesity become even more disturbing when weighing the health costs: Fully half of obese kids have a combination of high blood pressure, insulin resistance, unhealthy cholesterol, and other metabolic abnormalities.

Weight Loss

Vegetarianism is the *easiest and healthiest* way to lose weight. In a year-long study comparing Dean Ornish's vegetarian diet to the Weight Watchers program, the Zone diet, and the Atkins diet, the vegetarian diet showed the most weight loss (Dansinger et al., 2005). In general, the scientific literature has shown that dieters lose weight faster if they cut down on fat instead of carbohydrates, and as we have seen, vegetarians and vegans consume far less fat, especially saturated fat. Want to lose twenty pounds as effortlessly as humanly possible? Eliminate all animal products from your diet, and watch those pounds melt away.

Osteoporosis

Osteoporosis is a degenerative disease that causes people (disproportionately female) to lose bone mass as they age, which in turn leads to bone fractures and other painful injuries. Osteoporosis affects an estimated 75 million people in Europe, the United States, and Japan. One-third of women over fifty will experience these fractures, as will 20 percent of men. Thirty to 50 percent of women and 15 to 30 percent of men will suffer a fracture related to osteoporosis in their lifetime. Tragically, 40 percent of the people who break their hips never walk independently again, and 20 percent die within a year from related complications. The medical cost of treating osteoporosis is enormous and rising fast.

Fortunately, a vegetarian diet provides strong protection against this devastating disease. This is exciting news. Scientists think the reason for this phenomenon is that dietary protein increases the loss of calcium from bones and urinary calcium excretion, and this loss is far greater in individuals whose diets contain high levels of animal protein, *including dairy products*. Additionally, calcium is far more easily absorbed from plant sources than from animal sources. Let's look at some recent studies:

- In one research project, older women with a high dietary ratio of animal to vegetable protein suffered more rapid femoral neck bone loss and were at greater risk of hip fracture than those with a low ratio (Abelow et al. 1992).

- The Harvard Nurses Health Study, which included over 57,000 women, found women who consumed the most calcium from dairy products had almost double the rate of hip fractures compared to women who got the least amout of calcium from dairy sources.

- Another study found that vegetarian women between 50 and 89 years old lost 18 percent of their bone mass, while a control group of non-vegetarian women suffered a 35 percent bone loss (Sellmeyer et al., 2001).

- Additionally, osteoporosis-type hip fractures occur more frequently in countries with diets high in animal protein (Abelow et al., 1992).

Other Health Issues

Gallstones

Gallstones and kidney stones are composed of cholesterol, bile pigments, and calcium salts. Vegetarians are largely protected from these painful conditions, indeed, after controlling for age and weight, a meat eater was twice as likely to get gallstones as a vegetarian (Kratzer et al., 1997; Hughes & Norman, 1992).

Arthritis

The vegetarian diet has been shown to reduce both the pain and symptoms of rheumatoid arthritis with *dramatic* results, and again a plant-based diet often works better than our best medicine (Kjeldsen-Kragh et al., 1991; McDougall et al., 2002).

PMS

A vegetarian diet has been shown to greatly relieve both painful menstruation and premenstrual syndrome (Barnard et al., 2000).

> *“Biochemically, when a frightened animal knows it's going to be killed, a rush of adrenalin pulses through its body. After the kill, rigor mortis sets in, gases form, rot and putrefaction begin, and parasites have a feeding frenzy. Next it can be found on someone's dinner plate—yummy!”*
>
> —Spice Williams-Crosby, actress

The Hidden Horrors in Meat

Since they eat no meat, vegetarians consume none of the myriad of pesticides and other chemicals in meat. According to the U.S. Environmental Protection Agency, over 1 billion tons of pesticides are used in the United States every year and the use of pesticides in meat production is increasing throughout the world. (While the European Union has seen a slight decrease in the amount of pesticides used in meat production, this is only because they are using more toxic and stronger pesticides; the pesticide residue found on land, water, and in meat has not diminished.)

The agricultural chemical industry produces about 45,000 different pesticides based on approximately 600 active ingredients (EPA's pesticide program: FY 2004 annual report, 2004). Factory farm animals have very high concentrations of chemicals from a lifetime of being sprayed with these pesticides (usually to control flies and other pests) and from eating feed that has been sprayed on average eight times with these dangerous chemicals.

Beef has been found to carry sky-high levels of pesticide residues (Pesticide Data Program, Annual Summary Calendar Year 2002, 2004). Some of the more common chemicals found in animal fat are polychlorinated biphenyls (PCBs), dioxins and organochlorines, and persistent organic pollutants (POPs). These chemicals tend to accumulate in human and animal tissue, dangerously increasing in toxicity as they move up the food chain.

Farmers also pump animals full of hormones and growth stimulants to fatten them faster for slaughter. Happily vegetarians ingest none of these. Hormones such as Steer-oid, Ralgro, Compudose, and Synovex are used in thousands and thousands of feedlots throughout the world. Ingested through meat consumption, these chemical compounds can have a profound effect on human health even at the smallest doses, and no one knows the long-term effect of continuous ingestion.

Scientists report that the hormone residues found in meat can disrupt people's hormone balance, trigger developmental problems, interfere with reproductive systems, and lead to the development of cancer. Hormone residues are also thought to cause the early onset of puberty in girls; girls are reaching menses at younger and younger ages throughout the world. Alarmed by the mounting evidence against these practices, the European Union has banned all hormones used in meat production (Raloff 2002). Unfortunately, the United States and the rest of the world have yet to follow.

Antibiotics are poured into livestock, poultry and fish to promote growth and in a desperate effort to compensate for the unsanitary conditions, disease and resultant death found on factory farms. Just in the United States alone, humans use 2 million pounds of antibiotics annually to treat infections, while animals consume 3 million pounds. Another whopping 24.6 million pounds more of antibiotics are given to livestock to promote abnormal growth (Gorbach, 2001).

Because of this, antibiotics are losing their effectiveness on both people and animals worldwide; many illnesses no longer respond to antibiotics. The European Union has recently moved to ban seven antibiotics for use in growth promotion, while the European Commission Scientific Steering Committee proposed a ban on all growth promoters by 2006. (Nierenberg & Garcés, 2004). However, so far no action has been taken against this destructive practice anywhere in the world. It continues unabated.

> *"A dead cow or sheep lying in the pasture is recognized as carrion. The same sort of carcass dressed and hung up in a butcher's stall passes as food. Careful microscopic examination may show little or no difference … Both are swarming with colon germs and redolent with putrefaction."*
>
> —Dr. John Harvey Kellogg

Food Poisoning

Vegetarians are far less likely to be victims of food poisoning. With millions and millions of people suffering each year from food-borne illnesses, food poisoning is the most common disease in the world. An interesting note: Most people confuse food poisoning with "stomach flu," but diseases characterized by vomiting, diarrhea, and nausea, occasionally marked by a fever, are very often food poisoning. The actual number of food poisoning afflictions in the United States alone is staggering: According to the U.S. Centers for Disease Control, food-borne pathogens cause 76 million illnesses, 325,000 hospitalizations, and 5,000 deaths each year.

The United States Department of Agriculture estimates the annual economic loss from these illnesses at somewhere between $7 billion and $37 billion. Keep in mind these figures are comparable in the developed world, but *much higher* for developing countries. And meat, eggs, and dairy products are responsible for 95 percent of food poisoning (Hall, 1992).

> *"Lobsters roasted alive, pigs whipt to death, fowls sewed up, are testimonies to our outrageous luxury. Those who (as Seneca expresses it) divide their lives betwixt an anxious conscience and nauseated stomach, have a just reward of their gluttony in the diseases it brings with it."*
>
> —Alexander Pope, poet and writer

Mad Cow Disease

It is extremely rare for vegetarians to get variant Creutzfeldt-Jakob disease (vCJD), the human form of mad cow disease. Over 150 new cases of this disease appeared in England in recent years, and many more occurred in other countries. Unlike other parts of the world, the United States Department of Agriculture refuses to test an adequate number of cows for Bovine

Spongiform Encephalopathy (BSE or mad cow disease). Most countries test 50 percent of their cows, and some countries like Japan and Ireland test all of their cows. BSE appears in hundreds and hundreds of cows throughout the world, but as of this writing, the United States has reported only three cases.

Few people familiar with the subject believe this figure could possibly be accurate; many scientists fear that mad cow disease is far more prevalent in the U.S. meat supply, but because cows are brought to slaughter very young in the United States—usually at just under two years old—symptoms of BSE do not have enough time to manifest.

Still, every year an estimated 100,000 cows die of downer cow syndrome, a disease where cows appear fine one day and collapse and die the next in the same manner as BSE cows. Many scientists and agricultural experts suspect that the only reason the United States has so few cases of BSE is because we call it downer cow syndrome instead of mad cow disease or BSE. International concern over U.S. beef recently forced the USDA to tentatively agree to test 20,000 of these "downer" cows for BSE, but so far this has not happened.

Meanwhile, prions, the proteins that cause vCJD, have been found in an alarming percentage of the brains of people who died from Alzheimer's disease, and even in the tonsils of healthy people (Kelleher, 2004).

Some scientists are now theorizing that Alzheimer's is often mistaken for vCJD, as both diseases share many symptoms. Still, other scientists think the danger here is minimal, theorizing that if vCJD were a real danger to human health, we would have more cases of it. The incubation period of this terrible brain-wasting disease varies, but it can be twenty to thirty years, so no one knows for certain if a health crisis is looming in our future. Clearly, not enough is known about vCJD. More research needs to be done.

> *"You never hear anyone talk about mad tofu disease."*
>
> —John Robbins, author, *Diet For a New America*

OTHER WAYS TO LOSE YOUR MIND

Alzheimer's and other dementias continue to increase throughout the world and sadly, most people reading this have a close relative or family friend with Alzheimer's or dementia. An estimated 24 million people currently suffer some form of dementia, a number that is only expected to rise in the next twenty-five years with the world's aging populations. There is growing evidence that Alzheimer's disease and other dementias follow the familiar pattern of cardiovascular disease, and both are strongly linked to obesity and diabetes. The vegetarian diet offers substantial protection against these devastating old-age diseases. (Giem et al., 1993).

Other studies have shown that risk for

Alzheimer's is greater in people who consume diets high in cholesterol and saturated fats and low in fiber, vegetables, and fruits. Preliminary findings in still another study showed an increased incidence of dementia in people who consume a lot of meat compared with vegetarians. Additionally, predominantly vegetarian countries like India, where over 80 percent of the population does not eat beef, see a much lower percentage of their population afflicted by Alzheimer's, controlling, of course, for age of the population.

Nutrition, Vegetarian Myths, and the New V-Meats

Contrary to popular belief, vegetarians get plenty of protein. Indeed it is nearly impossible not to get enough protein in a *healthy* vegetarian diet of 2,000 calories a day. (One could consume a diet of gum drops and soda pop, that would be vegetarian and offer insufficient protein, but it wouldn't be healthy.) Nor is there any truth to the myth that one must mix certain vegetable proteins at meals to ensure proper nutrition. The whole idea that vegetarians had to mix proteins was based on the totally unsubstantiated *belief* of a 1950s doctor, and, inexplicably, this unsupported fancy took hold in the public consciousness.

Similarly, unlike meat eaters, vegetarians do not have to worry about getting too much protein. The average meat eater consumes 45 percent more protein a day than the daily recommendation. While no one knows the long-term effects of this, studies have shown that excessive animal protein can cause kidney damage, especially in older people. Excessive dietary protein has also been linked to diabetes (Diaz-Buxo, 1998), and osteoporosis (Cloutier & Barr, 2003).

> "*Vegetarians have the best diet. They have the lowest rate of coronary disease of any group in the country. They have a fraction of our heart attack rate and they have only 40 percent of our cancer rate.*"
>
> —William Castelli, M.D., director, Framingham Heart Study, the longest-running epidemiological study in medical history

New vegetarian meats make it easy to go without the real thing—vegetarian meats have evolved way past the dry oat-filled patty. There are now dozens of different kinds of vegetarian meat available: ground beef (an excellent substitute for hamburger in any recipe, especially Italian and Mexican recipes); chicken and beef patties, spicy or regular; hot dogs; veal cutlets; beef or chicken cutlets; chicken breasts or nuggets; bacon; pastrami; ham; sausage; baloney; turkey; even corn dogs!

There are vegetarian meats that are as tasty as their meat counterparts and some that are spicier and tastier. *Most have no cholesterol, no saturated fat, about one-fourth of the calories of regular meat, and many have over twice as much nutrition.*

Try the countless excellent dairy stand-ins as well. Soy milk has become a perfect milk alternative; except that soy milk is richer, sweeter, creamier, with no saturated fat or cholesterol, and significantly *more calcium and vitamins* per cup than milk.

> *"Human beings are not natural carnivores. When we kill animals to eat them, they end up killing us because their flesh, which contains cholesterol and saturated fat, was never intended for human beings, who are natural herbivores."*
>
> —Dr. William Roberts, editor-in-chief, *American Journal of Cardiology*

An Anatomy Lesson

While humans can digest flesh, and it is likely that our ancestors did consume *small* amounts of meat infrequently, our anatomy much more strongly resembles that of plant-eating creatures. Like all plant eaters the human colon is long and complex, and our intestines are ten to eleven times longer than our bodies. Meat eaters have a short and simple colon, and in order that putrid meats pass quickly through their bodies, their intestines are only three to six times longer than their bodies. Human saliva contains digestive enzymes; meat eaters' saliva does not. Our teeth resemble those of other plant eaters, with short and blunt canines, as opposed to long, sharp, and curved canines of the big meat eaters. Additionally, the meat our evolutionary ancestors consumed was wild game, which has less fat content than our modern domesticated meats.

The Only Drawback to Vegetarianism

> *"I am on the verge of 85 and still work as hard as ever. I have lived quite long enough and I am trying to die; but I simply cannot do it. A single beef-steak would finish me; but I cannot bring myself to swallow it. I am oppressed with a dread of living forever. That is the only disadvantage of vegetarianism."*
>
> —George Bernard Shaw, playwright

Bernard Shaw wittily articulates the conclusion of countless studies that demonstrate vegetarians live longer than meat eaters. The famous Loma Linda University study of 27,000 Seventh Day Adventists found a lower age-adjusted death rate for vegetarians than that of the general population. These vegetarians were less likely to die from heart disease, stroke, diabetes, and all cancers than the general population. Not only do vegetarians live longer, but those extra years will most likely be spent in excellent health!

> *"As long as there are slaughterhouses, there will be battlefields."*
>
> —Leo Tolstoy

FINALLY: THE BIG MEDICAL PICTURE

The medical costs just in the United States due to meat consumption were estimated to be $30 to 60 billion a year, based upon the higher prevalence of hypertension, heart disease, cancer, diabetes, gallstones, obesity, and food-borne illnesses among meat eaters as compared with vegetarians (Barnard et al., 1995). Because of skyrocketing medical costs in the last decade since this calculation, this figure is bound to be much higher today. Worldwide figures are incalculable. Chronic diseases are now the major cause of death and disability worldwide, but medical conditions associated with meat-laden diets, including cardiovascular diseases, diabetes, obesity, and cancer, now account for 59 percent of the 57 million deaths annually and 46 percent of the financial burden of disease.

> *"If we are reasonably sure of what our data from these studies are telling us, then why must we be reticent about recommending a diet which we know is safe and healthy? ...I personally have great faith in the public. We must tell them that a diet of roots, stems, seeds, flowers, fruit, and leaves is the healthiest diet and the only diet we can promote, endorse, and recommend."*
>
> —T. Colin Campbell, Ph.D., director,
> The China Health Study

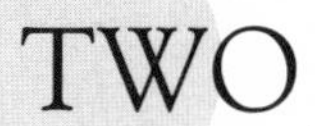

TWO

The Environmentally Conscious Vegetarian

"A reduction in beef and other meat consumption is the most potent single act you can take to halt the destruction of our environment and preserve our natural resources. Our choices do matter. What's healthiest for each of us personally is also healthiest for the life support system of our precious, but wounded planet."

—John Robbins, author, *Diet for a New America,* and President, EarthSave Foundation

The Damage Wrought by Meat Production

According to the United Nations Food and Agricultural Organization, 1.3 billion cattle, nearly 1 billion pigs, 1.8 billion sheep and goats, and over 15 billion chickens are raised and slaughtered for food every year, and each one of these animals produces waste. This is the earth's largest environmental problem. Animal waste is the number one source of water pollution in the world; it is responsible for over half of it. To bring the matter home, let's first look at some animal population statistics by country:

- The United States is raising over 94 million cows, 60 million pigs, 7 million sheep, and an astonishing 2 billion chickens at any given time.

- Canada keeps about 15 million cows, 15 million pigs, 1 million sheep, and 160 million chickens.

- China hosts about 107 million cows, 473 million pigs, 341 million sheep, and 4 billion chickens.

- Japan has 5 million cows, 10 million pigs, and 290 million chickens.

- Brazil has about 192 million cows, 33 million pigs, 7 million sheep, and 1.1 billion chickens.

- Argentina keeps about 51 million cows, 3 million pigs, 17 million sheep, and 95 million chickens.

- Mexico hosts 30 million cows, 18 million pigs,16 million sheep, and 540 million chickens.

- The United Kingdom keeps about 11 million cows, 5 million pigs, 36 million sheep, and 60 million chickens.

- France has 19 million cows, 15 million pigs, 10 million sheep, and 800 million chickens.

- Germany keeps about 13 million cows, 26 million pigs, 2 million sheep, and over 110 million chickens.

- The Netherlands hosts 4 million cows, 11 million pigs, 1 million sheep, and 100 million chickens.

- Denmark hosts 2.2 million cows, 13 million pigs, and about 17 million chickens.

- Finland keeps 1 million cows, 1 million pigs, and 6 million chickens.

- Sweden has 2 million cows, 2 million pigs, and 6 million chickens.

- New Zealand has 10 millions cows and 40 million sheep.

- Australia has 26 million cows, 3 million pigs, 95 million sheep, and 90 million chickens.

And You Thought Mount Everest Was Big!

Based on accepted manure rates per animal supplied by the United States Environmental Protection Agency's livestock manure handling overview, the worldwide amount of wastes from cattle is... *45 trillion* pounds of manure per year, a number that begins to sound like the calculation of the distance between stars, rather than piles of cow manure (Livestock Manure Handling on the Farm, 2002). Worldwide waste from pigs per year is...*6 trillion* pounds per year. Worldwide waste from sheep and goats is another *6 trillion* pounds per year. Worldwide waste from chickens reaches *1.5 trillion* pounds per year. A very small portion of these mountains of manure is used as fertilizer. The rest? Pollution.

- One study puts animal waste in the United States to between *2.4 trillion* to *3.9 trillion* pounds per year (Kellogg, 2000; Livestock Manure Handling on the Farm, 2002). Or put another way, the United States produces 15,000 pounds of manure per person, per year. This is 130 times the amount of waste produced by the entire human population of the United States (United States Department of Agriculture/ Environmental Protection Agency draft Unified National Strategy for Animal Feeding Operation, 1998). Yet unlike human waste, no animal waste is treated.

Let's look at this chart to see what is happening in individual countries:

Country	Total waste in billions of pounds per year	Population in millions	Pounds of animal feces per person per year
Argentina	1,840	39	47,179
Australia	1,100	20	37,377
Belgium	150	10	15,000
Brazil	6,840	183	37,377
Canada	590	32	18,437
China	7,400	1,330	5,563
Denmark	150	5	30,000
Finland	10	5	2,000
France	800	61	13,114
Germany	650	83	7,831
India	6,850	1,097	6,244
Japan	250	128	1,953
Mexico	1150	106	10,849
Netherlands	170	16	10,625
Norway	40	5	8,000
South Africa	570	45	12,670
Spain	430	41	10,490
Sweden	80	9	8,890
U.K.	480	60	8,000
U.S.A.	3,670	300	15,000

Here are some manure facts for each of the three major farm animals:

- A 1,000-cow dairy can produce approximately 120,000 pounds of waste per day. This is the functional equivalent of the amount of sanitary waste produced by a city of 20,000 people (Cook & Stanley, 1998).

- A 20,000-chicken factory produces about 2.4 million pounds of manure a year. Poultry factories are one of the fastest growing industries throughout Asia.

- One pig excretes nearly three gallons of waste per day, or 2.5 times the average human's daily total. One hog farm with 50,000 pigs in France produces more waste than the entire city of Los Angeles, and some pig farms are much larger.

- Indeed, hog farms of 150,000 animals are becoming commonplace. During the past fifteen years, the number of hog farms in the United States dropped from 600,000 to 157,000, yet the number of hogs remains almost the same. The same trend towards fewer livestock farms with larger numbers of animals and much larger waste disposal problems is seen throughout Europe, Japan, Korea, Taiwan, and China. For instance, in Japan, the average number of animals kept by a farm in 1992 was 25.7 times that of 1970.

Rivers and Waterways

Much of this pollution heads right into the world's waterways and rivers. According to the U.S. Environmental Protection Agency, the waste generated by hogs, chicken and cattle has polluted over 35,000 miles of rivers. The EPA estimates that this pollution from agriculture ruined or interfered with the aquatic life in, or public use of, a startling 173,629 river miles—25 percent of all river miles surveyed. Other scientists put the figure much higher; factory farms caused up to 70 percent of all water quality problems identified in rivers and streams (Cook & Stanley, 1998).

Pig farms are the worst: Manure and urine from many pig farms go into large, foul-smelling lagoons, and even a modest amount of rain can send the manure from these thousands of lagoons percolating directly into our precious water tables and spilling into our waterways. A North Carolina State University study concluded that fully half of the existing lagoons in the United States leak into water tables (Huffman & Westerman, 1995).

France, Germany, the Netherlands, and the United Kingdom are among the EU member countries facing severe agricultural water pollution problems as the result of factory farms (Scheierling, 1995).

Scientists in Japan have found that virtually all of the waterways in farming regions were heavily polluted by animal wastes (Harada, 1994).

These mountains of manure pose a much larger

threat to our waterways than urban runoff and industrial waste combined.

Groundwater

Perhaps the most alarming aspect of this water pollution shows up in the world's groundwater. Factory farms have contaminated groundwater in seventeen of the twenty-two states that report animal waste figures (USDA/EPA, 1998). Scientists investigating nitrate pollution found that groundwater in every one of the Chinese provinces of Beijing, Tianjin, Hebei, and Shandong was unfit for drinking due to livestock wastes; in Mexico more than half of groundwater sampled contained nitrate at levels above the safe limit; in Romania and Moldova, more than 35 percent of the sites sampled in the mid-1990s had nitrate concentrations higher than the health guideline (Sampat & Petersen, 2000). Nearly everywhere scientists look they find nitrate pollution infiltrating the world's precious freshwater lakes, rivers, and groundwater.

Coastal and Ocean Pollution

Factory farm pollution is the primary source of damage to coastal waters in North and South America, Europe, and Asia. Scientists report that over sixty percent of the coastal waters in the United States are moderately to severely degraded from factory farm nutrient pollution (Howarth et al., 2000). This pollution creates oxygen-depleted dead zones, which are huge areas of ocean devoid of aquatic life. One such zone in the Gulf of Mexico now covers a 20,000 square-kilometer section of water, an area approximately half the size of the Netherlands. (Howarth et al., 2000).

Some of this pollution or agricultural runoff triggers harmful algae blooms (HAB), commonly called red or brown tides, which often destroy fisheries (European initiative on harmful algal blooms, 2002). The price tag for HABs is astronomical: The National Oceanic and Atmospheric Administration (NOAA) conservatively estimated that HABs cost the United States 1 billion dollars a year, and this is just for ocean fisheries (Spinrad, 2005). For instance, from 1995 to just 1998, 200 manure-related fish kills resulted in the death of 13 million fish just in the United States. In a particularly bad spill, 25 million gallons of waste from an eight-acre lagoon in North Carolina killed 10 million fish in the New River and closed 364,000 acres of coastal wetlands to shell fishing (Singer, 2002).

Similar costs accrue from fresh water HABs around the world as well. Occurring wherever fresh water and meat production mix, freshwater HABs are becoming more costly every year: These freshwater HABs in Australia alone cost between $180 million and $240 million each year (LWRRDC, 2000). These poisonous blooms occasionally become so toxic as to cause people's deaths, either by direct contact or by the ingestion of poisoned fish.

Here's the frightening fact: Throughout the world

HABs now occur more often, cover ever larger areas of water, and last longer. (European initiative on harmful algal blooms, 2002).

Diseases

These mountains of animal waste are home to countless disease-causing pathogens, such as Salmonella, E. coli, Cryptosporidium, and fecal coliform, which can be ten to 100 times more concentrated than in human waste. More than forty diseases can be transferred to humans through manure (Marks, 2001).

> *"Five tons of poop apiece is just the residue of eating 100 million cattle, 103 million hogs, 300 million turkeys, and nearly nine billion chickens per year, virtually all of whom live and die in conditions that would be prosecutable cruelty if inflicted on a cat, a dog, a horse, or a parrot. Whether you care about animals or just about poop, appropriate action begins with giving up meat."*
>
> —Merritt Clifton, author, animal rights activist

Global Warming

Vegetarianism combats global warming in meaningful ways. As we all know, global warming threatens the world's climates and ecologies. This danger is caused by the pollution from burning fossil fuels: coal, gas and oil. The main culprit is carbon dioxide, but nitrous oxide, methane, manmade CFCs, and ozone all contribute as well. While scientists still debate the rate of global warming and its consequences, they agree that global warming is a reality and a looming menace. The vegetarian diet produces far less of these treacherous greenhouse gases. Here are the numbers:

- A tremendous amount of energy is used to transport food throughout the world. A colossal 70 percent of the world's agriculture resources are consumed in meat production. Petroleum is used in the raising, harvesting, and transporting of vast amounts of crops fed to farm animals, as well as the transportation of these animals, the processing of the animals into meat, and the transportation of the meat to the consumer.

  According to the U.S. Department of Transportation, agricultural products are transported 566 billion ton-miles within United States borders each year, constituting more than 20 percent of all United States commodity transports. These figures are similar in parts of Asia and all of Europe.

  The global economy is a tremendous trigger to the skyrocketing amounts of petroleum used in meat production. For instance, the European Union imports most of its animal feed from South America; the United States exports beef to Japan; New Zealand sends lamb to the Middle

East, the European Union, and North America. In fact, it takes a massive three times more fossil fuel to produce a meat-centered diet than a plant-centered diet (Singer, 2002). Or put another way, the yearly beef consumption of the average family of four in the United States requires over 260 gallons of fossil fuel, creating as much carbon dioxide as the average car emits in six months of normal operation (Rifkin, 1992).

- Livestock accounts for nearly 25 percent of total methane emissions (Methane: Sources and Emissions, 2004) Methane is the second biggest contributor to global warming.

- Livestock also accounts for 7 percent of all nitrous oxide emissions worldwide (Fritschel & Mohan, 1999).

The Double Whammy: Deforestation and Global Warming

Meat production causes deforestation, which then contributes to global warming. Trees convert carbon dioxide into oxygen, and the destruction of forests around the world to make room for grazing cattle furthers the greenhouse effect. The Food and Agricultural Organization of the United Nations reports that the annual rate of tropical deforestation has increased from 9 million hectares in 1980 to 16.8

million hectares in 1990, and unfortunately this destruction has accelerated in the last decade and a half. (Please note that *one* hectare equals 10,000 square meters, or 2.471 acres). By 1994, a staggering 200 million hectares of rainforest had been destroyed in South America just for cattle (Gussow, 1994).

In the ensuing twelve years, this rate of destruction had not abated. According to the Center for International Forestry Research, an Indonesia-based NGO, in Brazil alone the rainforest loss in 2002–2003 is expected to exceed 25,000 square kilometers, a plot the size of Uruguay. The cattle population has exploded in the Amazon, from 26 million in 1990 to 57 million in 2002. Likewise much of the deforestation in Central America, Brazil, and Indonesia results in farmland that generates the feed used in European factory farms. To put the numbers in perspective: the average car emits 3 kg/day of CO_2, but clearing enough rainforest to produce beef for one hamburger results in an output of 75 kg of CO_2. In this way, eating one pound of hamburger does as much damage as driving your car for more than three weeks (Boyan, 2005).

> *“Carl Pope could probably affect the world more by being a vegetarian than through his job as president of the Sierra Club.”*
>
> —Jennifer Horsman

Species Extinction Explained

Livestock pollution and deforestation contribute to species extinction, which is also a tragic global phenomenon. Loss of tropical rainforest has a far more profound effect than the mere destruction of aesthetically beautiful areas. It has been estimated that without the effects of deforestation, the world loses ten to fifteen species a year, but some experts estimate that a startling 40,000 species are lost each year due to deforestation.

If the current rate of deforestation continues, the world's rainforests will vanish within fifty years—causing unknown effects on global climate and eliminating the majority of plant and animal species on the planet. According to a 1997 report of endangered species in the southwestern United States by the Fish and Wildlife Service, half the species studied were threatened by cattle ranching. This becomes a much larger problem as meat production increases in the developing world where much of the world's biodiversity exists.

> "*The impact of countless hooves and mouths over the years has done more to alter the type of vegetation and land forms of the West than all the water projects, strip mines, power plants, freeways, and sub-division developments combined.*"
>
> —Philip Fradkin, in *Audubon,*
> National Audubon Society, New York

More Air Pollution

It doesn't stop there. Agricultural meat production generates even more air pollution. As manure decomposes, it releases over 400 volatile organic compounds, many of which are extremely harmful to human health (Halverson, 2001).

Let's look at the major by-product of animal wastes—nitrogen. Nitrogen changes to ammonia as it escapes into the air, and this is a major source of acid rain. Worldwide, livestock produces over 30 million tons of ammonia (Agriculture: Towards 2015/30 technical interim report, 2000). Just the pig and poultry industries produce 6.9 million tons of nitrogen per year. A small farming state like North Carolina releases 186 tons of ammonia into the air *each day* (Halverson, 2001). Germany's livestock emits about 750 thousand tons a year, the Netherlands 181 thousand tons a year. Over half of acid rain is caused by ammonia emissions from factory farms. This situation keeps worsening. Traces of pure urine have actually been found in rain water! (Halverson, 2001).

Hydrogen sulfide is another chemical released from animal waste. This chemical smells like rotten eggs in low concentrations and can cause irreversible neurological damage even at these low levels (Halverson 2001). In 1998, the National Institutes of Health reported that nineteen people died as a result of hydrogen sulfide emissions from manure pits.

Additionally, people who reside within a twenty-mile radius of a hog farm suffer numerous ill effects.

These individuals experience greatly increased rates of respiratory disease and asthma, and they claim that the stench permeates everything from their homes to their clothes.

Clair describes living near a pig farm in North Dakota:

> We lived about fifteen miles from a large hog operation. Most days the stench was unimaginable. We couldn't sit on our porch or in the backyard, and the kids got so that they didn't want to go outside to play. No matter what I tried, I couldn't get it off our clothes. My youngest got teased at school, and well, imagine going to church carrying the faint but discernable scent of pig manure.
>
> Our property value plummeted; we probably couldn't give our house away, and we had no choice really but to sue the owner, which turned out to be a big corporation. But what got to me most was the idea of the pigs themselves. The workers all wore masks to protect their lungs, but no one cared about the pigs. The air burns their lungs and causes all kinds of respiratory diseases, and so they have to pump 'em full of antibiotics just to keep them alive.
>
> The whole thing is not right....

Ocean Fisheries

Vegetarians help to preserve the ocean's fisheries. Fishing provides a livelihood and food security for 200 million people, especially in the developing world, and one of five people on this planet depends on fish as a primary source of protein. Unfortunately, seafood has never been more popular in the industrialized world. Making matters worse, fully one-third of all harvested fish is fed to livestock. New technology—sophisticated sonar equipment and impossibly large nets—have allowed us to tremendously increase the exploitation of countless marine species.

The World Conservation Union lists well over 1,000 different fish species that are threatened or endangered. According to the United Nations Food and Agriculture Organization's (FAO) estimate, over 70 percent of the world's fish species are either fully exploited or depleted. For instance, commercial fish populations of cod, hake, haddock, and flounder have fallen by as much as 95 percent in the north Atlantic. On top of everything else, thousands upon thousands of other animal species also depend upon the ocean fisheries in a complex web of vital ecology, and too often diminishing numbers of one species results in the loss of many others. For instance, for each pound of shrimp consumed by people, four or more pounds of other marine life are caught and killed in the by-catch.

> *"No single activity or combination of activities has contributed more to the deterioration of plant and animal life than the nibbling mouths and pounding hooves of livestock."*
>
> —Richard Rabkin and Jacob Rabkin, authors

Soil Erosion

In the last two decades there has been a growing appreciation of the threat to European, Asian, Africa, and North, South and Central America soils as a result of intensification of agriculture and overgrazing. In Central and South America, two-thirds of the richest farm land is used as pasture for cattle, as well as all of the farm land lining rivers. Most of this meat does not feed the people of the region—rather it is exported abroad, mostly to the United States. The poorer farmers farm hillsides or cut down more forests, both of which also contribute to massive soil erosion. Soon these smaller farmers completely exploit the soil and are obliged to move on, carrying their destructive habits with them. (Soils, Farming, Forests, UNA-Canada, 2002).

Similarly, the number of people and animals skyrocketed in Africa, and overgrazing in some countries is thought to exceed the carrying capacity of the range by 100 percent, leading to massive soil erosion, water pollution, and desertification (Soils, Farming, Forests, UNA-Canada, 2002). Likewise the United States and Europe lose several billion tons of topsoil each year from cropland and grazing land—and 84 percent of this erosion is caused by livestock agriculture. While this soil is theoretically a renewable resource, we are losing it much faster than we are able to replace it. It takes 100 to 500 years to produce one inch of topsoil, but due to livestock grazing and feeding, farming areas can lose up to six inches of topsoil a year.

> *"One friend reports having a flash of understanding when he stood by a fence that separated grazed and ungrazed portions of the same creek bed. One side was lush and verdant. The other side looked like the face of the moon."*
>
> —Donald M. Peters, in the *Arizona Republic*

Land Resources

Livestock production affects a startling 70 to 85 percent of the land area of the United States, United Kingdom, and European Union. That includes the public and private rangeland used for grazing, as well as the land used to produce the crops that feed the animals. By comparison, urbanization—which concerns a good many people—only affects 3 percent of the United States land area, slightly more for the European Union and the United Kingdom. These figures vary somewhat in Asia and South and Central America, but the point remains: Meat production consumes the world's land resources.

"Animal factories are one more sign of the extent to which our technological capacities have advanced faster than our ethics. We plow under habitats of other animals to grow hybrid corn that fattens our genetically engineered animals for slaughter. We make free species extinct and domestic species into bio-machines. We build cruelty into our diet."

—Peter Singer and Jim Mason,
authors, *The Way We Eat*

GRAIN RESOURCES

The world's cattle consume an amount of food equivalent to the calorie requirements of 8.7 billion people. *Read that sentence again.* Seventy percent of the grain grown in the United States is consumed by livestock. The wealthy nations feed more grain to their livestock than the people of India and China (more than one-third of the human race) consume directly. Two-thirds of the United States' agricultural exports go to feed livestock rather than hungry people. We have a choice of continuing to pour our grain into meat production or using it to feed the burgeoning hungry of our human populations.

"To be an environmentalist who happens to eat meat is like being a philanthropist who doesn't happen to give to charity."

—Howard Lyman, author, *Mad Cowboy*

Precious Water Resources

Half of all fresh water worldwide is used for thirsty livestock. The number is much higher for the western part of the United States and other areas of intense cattle and pig farming. Producing eight ounces of beef requires an unimaginable 25,000 liters of water, or the water necessary for one pound of steak equals the water consumption of the average household for a year (Lyman & Merzer, 1997).

> *"Under the leadership of Dr. King, I became totally committed to nonviolence, and I was convinced that nonviolence meant opposition to killing in any form. I felt the commandment "Thou Shall Not Kill" applied to human beings not only in their dealings with each other but in their practice of killing animals for food or sport. Animals and humans suffer and die alike. Violence causes the same pain, the same spilling of blood, the same stench of death, the same arrogant, cruel, and brutal taking of life."*
>
> —Dick Gregory, comedian, civil rights activist

Wildlife

In the United States, the government spends $10 million each year to kill an estimated 100,000 wild animals, including coyotes, foxes, bobcats, badgers, bears, and mountain lions just to placate ranchers who don't want these animals killing their livestock. The cost far outweighs the damage to livestock that these predators cause.

In the western United States, grazing cattle has pushed out countless wild animals from habitat areas. Worldwide, deforestation takes a huge toll on thousands and thousands of wild animal species.

Some wildlife biologists theorize that humankind's rapacious hunger for meat production and its drain on land, forested areas, and water resources will effectively eliminate all wild land mammals from earth in fifty years. The single exception? Rats are probably the only mammal that will manage to survive with us.

THE AMAZING VEGETARIAN DIFFERENCE

The vegetarian diet uses *far fewer* resources than a meat diet. First, just look at what Worldwatch Institute estimates one pound of steak from a steer raised in a feedlot costs: five pounds of grain, a whopping 2,500 gallons of water, the energy equivalent of a gallon of gasoline, and about 35 pounds of topsoil.

Additionally, farmland put to use for a vegetarian diet yields so much more than that which supports a meat diet. For instance, one acre of land can produce 40,000 pounds of potatoes, 30,000 pounds of carrots, 50,000 pounds of tomatoes, or 250 pounds of beef (Lyman & Merzer, 1997).

> "*Earth is generous with her provisions, and her sustenance is very kind; she offers, for your table, food that requires no bloodshed and no slaughter.*"
>
> —Ovid

The vegetarian diet fits the very definition of sustainability: 33 percent of our nation's raw materials and fossil fuels go into livestock destined for slaughter. When everyone jumps on the vegetarian bandwagon, only 2 percent of our resources will go to the production of food (Robbins, 1987).

> "*It seems disingenuous for the intellectual elite of the first world to dwell on the subject of too many babies being born in the second- and third-world nations while virtually ignoring the over-population of cattle and the realities of a food chain that robs the poor of sustenance to feed the rich a steady diet of grain-fed meat.*"
>
> —Jeremy Rifkin, author, *Beyond Beef: The Rise and Fall of the Cattle Culture*, and president of the Greenhouse Crisis Foundation

Going vegetarian can positively affect world hunger; it is a great humanitarian act. The World Health Organization estimates that, in 2006, 20 million people will die of malnutrition worldwide, and over half of these people will be children. Lester Brown of the Overseas Development Council calculates that if Americans reduced their meat consumption by only 10 percent per year, it would free at least 12 million tons of grain for human consumption—or enough to feed 60 million people. The food spent on animal production, if properly distributed, could end malnutrition and hunger throughout the world (Singer, 2002).

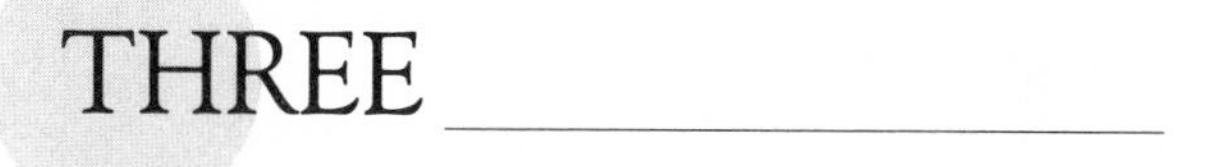

The Compassionate Vegetarian

> *"Those who, by their purchases, require animals to be killed have no right to be shielded from the slaughterhouse or any other aspect of the production of the meat they buy. If it is distasteful for humans to think about, what can it be like for the animals to experience it?"*
>
> —Dr. Peter Singer, professor of philosophy, Princeton University

Vegetarians include animals in the circle of their compassion. Animals are sentient creatures; they suffer fear, anxieties, and pain just as they experience love, contentment, and joy. The vegetarian philosophy regarding animals is both profound and simple: It is wrong to make animals suffer and to kill them inhumanely. Vegetarians do not participate in the abuse and inhumane killing of the cows, pigs, sheep, goats, or chickens that are raised and slaughtered every year. This is the great blessing of being a vegetarian, and the very best reason to become one.

> “*The question is not, can they reason? Nor, can they talk? But can they suffer?*”
>
> —Jeremy Bentham,
> philosopher, theologian

Vegetarians hold this truth to be self-evident: There is no moral distinction between bringing suffering and death upon an animal with your own hands and perpetrating it by paying someone to do it for you.

> “*As I cannot kill, I cannot authorize others to kill. Do you see? If you are buying from a butcher you are authorizing him to kill—to kill helpless, dumb creatures which neither you nor I could kill ourselves.*”
>
> —Paul Troubetzkoy, sculptor

The process of becoming a vegetarian acts like a spark to consciousness, and as you journey down this path, you become mindful of the connection between the living, breathing creature and the package of meat or fish neatly wrapped in the supermarket.

"All the arguments to prove man's superiority cannot shatter this hard fact: In suffering the animals are our equals."

—Dr. Peter Singer

Farm animals face the harshest of lives. Corporations have taken over the world's farms, and assembly line production on factory farms is the cruel means by which we turn the living animal into food. The sheer quantity of meat demanded by consumers prohibits any and all humane treatment, even the smallest act of kindness. Each and every one of these billions of animals is born into suffering, a suffering that does not end until the day that the animal is slaughtered. Because of the staggering number of animals involved, it is literally impossible to grasp the magnitude of the cruelty involved in meat eating.

"Man has an infinite capacity to rationalize his rapacity, especially when it comes to something he wants to eat."

—Cleveland Amory, founder, Fund for Animals

Lisa in Montana describes the contented lives of her chickens in a lively portrait that contrasts sharply to the tortured existence of factory farm chickens:

> My chickens are amazing and very curious creatures—I have nineteen. They love attention, but

are very independent. Some are feisty, bossy, or shy; some are bold as all get out (chasing back my dog, Cody); and some are wanderers. I might find one roosting in a tree half a mile away. I have four who come to the sound of their names. They each have a special set of friends that they hang with, and each bird seems to know her place in the scheme of her small chicken world.

They have a nice coop and a huge yard to peck and scratch in and dust bathe. When I walk around it, they follow me like little sheep, frantically swarming my legs as I toss stale bread, fruit, or veggies. Inside the coop, their hay-filled roosts line the walls. They like the nests made just so, protected from the curious eyes of the other chickens, and they will only lay where and when no one else is sitting. There are always a few who decide to sit and stay over the eggs in a particular nest. I call them the " stay-at-home moms."

When I read about the chickens on a factory farm, I sat down and wept.

The Lowly Broiler Chicken

Factory farm broiler chickens (table chickens) never know a moment's peace or contentment. From the day the baby chicks hatch, they are confined in windowless sheds, kept there in the most crowded conditions imaginable. The noise—desperate squawks and squeals—is deafening. Food, water, and the growth promoting antibiotics that make them mushroom out five or more pounds in just over a month are all dispensed from hoppers hanging from the roof. In most parts of the world none of the birds sees natural light until the day they are taken out to be killed. During the first few weeks of their short lives, they are often subjected to light for twenty-three hours a day in hopes that their systems will be fooled into signaling them to eat more. Their very biology is not safe from intrusion and abuse. The birds' lives are spent in a continuous state of distress, confusion, and discomfort. Additionally:

- Due to genetic manipulation and the content of their feed, 90 percent of broiler chickens have trouble walking (Marcus, 2000). Many birds' fragile legs just collapse from their unnatural weight.

- The worst of the birds' ordeal is, hands down, the foul air. Because of chronic overcrowding, the air the chickens breathe is full of ammonia, microorganisms, and dust from their droppings. The ammonia is so intense as to scorch their lungs; each breath brings discomfort. After pumping hormones into their food to make these simple creatures grow unnaturally quickly, the chicken farmer must now pump the chickens full of antibiotics to keep them alive. People who live around the sheds are instructed to stay as far away from them as possible; the intense pollution is a hazard to human health as well.

- Due to chronic overcrowding, feather plucking and cannibalism are common in the sheds, so chickens must have their beaks removed. This is a gruesome process in which the baby bird is placed against a searing hot guillotine that slices off the beak. On average, 30 percent of the birds—billions of animals—are seriously injured at this point. These injuries are often so severe that the bird, suffering from chronic pain, does not eat enough and fails to thrive. Injured and ill birds are never removed from the shed, and instead are left to die slow and painful deaths.

- A chicken's normal life span is seven years, but the broiler chicken's is only seven weeks.

> “*But for the sake of some little mouthful of flesh we deprive a soul of the sun and light, and of that proportion of life and time it had been born into the world to enjoy.*”
>
> —Plutarch

Billions upon Billions of Eggs

In egg production, the male chicks are destroyed on the day they are born—250 million of them meet this fate every year in the U.S. alone. Some companies gas the baby birds, but often they are stuffed into plastic bags, where they suffocate beneath the weight of the other sacks tossed over them. Others are ground up *while still alive*, to become food for their sisters.

> *"The argument that a group of individuals is 'all alike' has been used throughout human history as a justification for the oppression of that group. If all individuals are alike, then they become impersonal and killing them seems less wrong or horrendous. Chickens, whether intelligent or stupid, individual or identical, are sentient beings. They feel pain and experience fear. This, in itself, is enough to make it wrong to cause them pain and suffering."*
>
> —Jennifer Raymond, author, *The Peaceful Palate*

Laying hens also have a merciless, joyless existence. The birds' cages, called battery cages, are cruelly small. Four or five mature birds are placed in a 12-by-20-inch cage—about the size of one and a half pieces of letterhead-sized paper. Imagine that! The bird is unable to spread her wings. The noise level seems shot straight from hell. This will house the hen for as long as she lives; the tortures of the cage will be all she knows. It is troubling to note that in scientific experiments, whenever chickens were presented with the choice between freedom with no food and a cage with food, the chickens chose freedom. Additionally:

- The floors of these cages tilt forward slightly to force the eggs onto a conveyer belt and the angle is very uncomfortable for the birds' feet.

- Millions of birds' feet get stuck and begin to actually grow around the wire cage—an unimaginably painful process.

- In the battery cage, laying hens cannot stand comfortably. Even when one or two settle for a moment, the other birds are still in motion, so the comfortable position lasts only seconds.

- The constant jostling and bumping into each other leads to plucking; caged laying hens then lose their feathers. Their skin begins to rub raw against the cages, resulting in festering sores. Fear, feather loss, and pain are all part of the same syndrome, a syndrome that reflects a sad life indeed—and one suffered billions and billions of times a year.

> *"If you can't conceive of beating an animal, you shouldn't conceive of eating an animal."*
>
> —Natalie Merchant,
> songwriter, musician

Both laying hens and broiler chickens face a gruesome end. The doors are finally flung open, and workers, wearing masks to protect their lungs, grab the birds and stuff them, squawking in pain and terror, six or seven to a transport box. The boxes are stacked on top of each other. The creatures may receive no food or water during this time, which can last for days.

> *"If you are interested in preventing animal suffering, the first thing you should give up is eggs and milk, because the animals who produce those foods lead the most unhappy lives."*
>
> —Cesar Chavez

Finally, upon reaching the slaughterhouse, the birds are taken out of the box and one by one hung upside down on a conveyer belt. They are brought, still crying out in fear and pain, to the place where their throats are slit. Because of the frantic, impossible pace of killing at the slaughterhouses, many chickens are still alive when tossed into the feather-removal tanks of scalding hot water.

Chickens are sadly exempt from most nations' humane slaughter laws. These billions of chickens are killed every year outside any regulatory and humane consideration whatsoever. While the slaughter itself is horrifying, at least their joyless lives are over—the only mercy humans have shown them.

A Billion Doomed Wilburs

"I never liked killing pigs. I never did. And after Babe, I absolutely refuse to eat a pig."

—Oprah Winfrey

Roughly one billion pigs are raised and killed every year; each animal is a reason to become a vegetarian.

- These lively, sociable and intelligent creatures' lives are mercilessly short and full of nothing but intense suffering. The pigs' lives are so dismal that they often die for no known reason beyond the stress of their intense confinement (Halverson, 2000).

- Pigs are born and suckled in a small, enclosed "farrowing" unit. They are brought to slaughter weight in an indoor feed unit—typically by six months. Their entire lives are spent indoors, on either hard, concrete flooring or slatted wood flooring, both of which cause foot, hoof, and leg injuries. For the vast majority of pigs, not once do they see the sunlight, or feel the warmth of the sun on their backs, or taste fresh air.

- However, stress, boredom, and intense crowding are the least of their problems. The greatest abuse is the foul air the pigs are forced to breathe. As we have seen, animal waste creates ammonia, methane, and a number of other pollutants. The more animals, the more waste, the more pollution. The ammonia and methane destroy the pigs' lungs, scorching them with every breath to the degree that over 80 percent of United States pigs have pneumonia upon slaughter. (Horrigan et al., 2002).

The European Union, Japan, Mexico, and South America show similar figures. Like the chicken farmers, pig farmers must drug their animals with antibiotics in order to keep the pigs alive when suffering from these chronic respiratory diseases. Humans wear masks when feeding and watering the pigs, but of course the pigs have no such luxury.

- The smells hint at the agony brought by breathing this pollution day and night. Keep in mind the fact that pigs have a far more acute sense of smell than people and a strong inclination for cleanliness.

- Some unfortunate female pigs will not make it to slaughter in the first half year of their lives. Instead they will be put into pig production. Pig farmers think of these sows as pig-producing machines. They place the creatures in small stalls called gestation crates; and if that weren't bad enough, they sometimes keep the animals tethered within these cramped spaces.

For the rest of her life, the pig cannot move in any direction. From a study by G. Cronin as quoted in Peter Singer's *Animal Liberation,* here is an observation of how sows behave when first put in a stall with a tether:

> "The sows threw themselves violently backwards, straining against the tether[s]. Sows thrashed their heads about as they twisted and turned in their struggle to free themselves. Often loud screams were emitted and occasionally individuals crashed bodily against the side boards of the tether stalls."

According to Singer, these violent attempts to escape can go on for as long as three hours. Afterwards a sow will lie motionless quietly grunting and whining, for long periods. The sows show other typical signs of stress, such as gnawing at the bars of their stalls and chewing when there is nothing to chew.

That's it, for the rest of her life she will produce baby pigs.

- Industry authorities estimate that approximately 20 percent of these pigs die prematurely from exhaustion and stress due to the severe confinement and inhumane breeding schedules (Halverson, 2000). This practice of placing sows in gestation crates is so egregiously inhumane that it is now banned in the United Kingdom and Sweden, and will be illegal in the European Union in 2013. One state in the United States, Florida, has also banned it by popular vote.

- Once the piglets are born, they will be allowed to stay with their mother for one week before they are taken away. The trend is to shorten even this brief period. As anyone with an ounce of sense realizes, one of the cruelest things to do to a mother is to separate her from her offspring.

Dairy Cows

Here is a description of the nature of cows, in contrast to their lives on a factory farm:

> In an ideal situation, cows lead peaceful and contented lives. Cattle are extremely social; herds can form with up to 300 animals, individual cows can recognize about 100 individuals. They show a distinct preference for some friends (mothers and daughters seem especially close), while avoiding others.
>
> They moo to each other frequently and in this way keep contact even when out of each other's sight. Like horses and other herd animals, they also communicate through a series of different body positions and facial expressions.
>
> Cows are especially attached to their calves. If a

> cow finds herself on the opposite side of a fence from her calf, she will become agitated and call fearfully. Desperate to be reunited with her baby, she will stay by the fence through all kinds of weather, hunger, and even thirst. The strength of this bond continues even after the calf is fully grown. Mother cows have been known to travel up to seven miles in order to be reunited with their calves.
>
> Cattle have near panoramic vision, which allows them to watch for humans and other predators. Like us, they can see in color, except red. Their sense of smell is acute; they can detect scents more than six miles away. Cattle seem to love the moonlight, and they appear to remain busy for longer periods when the moon is full. The life span of cattle averages 20 to 25 years.

Nowadays, dairy cows are little more than living milk machines. They are often raised indoors in individual stalls with just enough room to stand and lie down with artificial lighting sixteen hours a day—temperature and food are controlled, without regard to comfort for the sole purpose of making the largest possible amount of milk.

- The dairy cows' calves are taken away usually within a day of being born. This causes unimaginable agony to the animals. The new mothers moan pitiably upon the forced separation.

- From the day of separation forward, the cow will be milked two or three times a day for about ten months. After the third month she is made pregnant again, and the cycle starts anew. A dairy cow typically lasts no more than four years before her milk production drops enough to make her more profitable as hamburger or dog food. Off to the slaughterhouse she goes.

> "*It should not be thought that animals go meekly and willingly into the death chambers—they are filled with terror and resist strongly.*"
>
> —Geoffrey Rudd, author, *Vegetarians and the Bible*

The Tragic Lives of Male Calves

All animals suffer horribly in our factory farms, but none more than the male calves on their way to becoming veal. In order to provide people with pale and tender meat, the calf is subjected to the most stressful and unnatural of lives. The only mercy is that it is short.

- The calf's suffering begins as he is ripped from the comfort of his mother. Scared and confused, missing his mom, he is placed in a small wooden box—measuring less than two feet wide and less than five feet long. This space is so cramped that he is unable to turn around or lie down—a source of constant frustration and discomfort. On the slatted floor, the calf is in a perpetual state of distress. Veal producers do not want the baby calf to develop muscles or burn calories (feed is expensive!), so they never allow the calf to leave this small, tight, and extremely uncomfortable space.

- He never sees the sun or breathes fresh air. He can never even feel a moment's peace as he consumes an extremely unnatural diet forced upon him by the farmer. In an effort to keep his flesh pale, the calf is almost completely deprived of iron. Farmers refuse to give the calves water even, thus forcing them to drink more of their special feed. The tight space prevents the desperate calves from even turning to lap up their urine, which they do if given any chance. That's how desperate they are to score a trickle of iron or appease their relentless thirst.

- The poor creature wants only its mother, to suck and to find a comfortable place to stand or lie down, but he is denied these simple things. Indeed, veal producers often keep the calves in darkness in order to reduce their movements even further. So extreme is the cruelty involved in producing veal that veal producers throughout the world often have a hard time finding vets who will treat their animals.

"As we talked of freedom and justice one day for all, we sat down to steaks. I am eating misery, I thought, as I took my first bite. I spit it out."

—Alice Walker, author, *The Color Purple*

LUCKY CATTLE?

Some cattle are the luckiest of all the farm animals; they typically enjoy six glorious months of freedom—of smelling the wind, feeling the sun and rain, and grazing to their hearts' content. After roaming free for six to eight months, they are shipped to the feedlot and here their misery begins. They are not caged at the feedlot, but they do spend the next eight months on barren dirt. They become victims of the elements, as few farmers provide shade during the hot summer months or warmth during cold winters. Cows want only to graze and chew their cud, but these simple pleasures are denied them in order to force them to eat the concentrated feed designed to fatten them quickly. Manure piles up; the smells are foul; and cows are far more sensitive to this olfactory assault than humans.

- Life on the range is good, except for harsh weather conditions, and the interruptions of painful procedures —castration, branding, and dehorning—all performed without benefit of anesthetics.

  Contrary to popular belief, horns are not insensitive material like fingernails; they contain nerves and blood vessels, both of which are cut in the removal process. Everything changes with the stressful transport to the feedlot. Here cattle face extreme crowding.

> *"As the trucks rolled by, I saw the cows and sheep in those trucks being transported. One could only see their eyes through the slits in the trucks, and it struck me that that was very much like the scene out of the Holocaust period of Jews being transported in cattle trucks to their fate. During the Holocaust, I am sure that the German people were aware that Jews and others were being treated in the most horrific way. They may not have known all the details, but they must have known something, but they didn't want to think about it. And I think today, we also don't want to think about the way in which animals are being treated. So there is a parallel in terms of our desire not to reflect on what is really happening."*
>
> —Rabbi Dan Cohn-Sherbok, author, professor

To the Slaughterhouses

The transportation of farm animals to the slaughterhouse is perhaps the cruelest aspect of their ordeal. The pigs, cattle, calves, sheep, and lambs board the trucks or train cars in a state of fear and confusion. Trips take between forty-eight and seventy-two hours. For cattle heading to a feedlot, the trip is sometimes even longer—and the creatures are often deprived of food, water, and rest for the duration. The animals cannot speak to tell us of their pain, but their worn-out bodies paint a sorrowful picture. Farmers call it "shrinkage"—the amount of weight an animal loses during transportation from stress and nutritional deprivation. It is not uncommon for cows to lose 10 percent of their body weight from dehydration during transportation.

- An animal's death in transit is not an easy one, nor is it uncommon. Countless creatures freeze to death during winter, or perish of thirst and heatstroke in the summer. Many often simply die from the unbearable stress of the process.

> "*You have just dined, and however scrupulously the slaughterhouse is concealed in the graceful distance of miles, there is complicity.*"
>
> —Ralph Waldo Emerson

At the Slaughterhouses

Meatpacking plants have the highest nonfatal injury and illness incidence rates among industries worldwide, primarily due to the pressure to move far too many animals too quickly through the slaughterhouse. Furthermore, because slaughterhouse supervisors are under a lot of pressure to report low injury rates, injury log falsification is rampant; many experts think the actual rates are much higher than those reported. One can scarcely imagine a worse job:

Slaughterhouse workers have astronomical rates of alcoholism and domestic violence (Eisnit, 1997). There is a heavy physical cost to the large-scale slaughter of animals, and—understandably—slaughterhouse workers exhibit the highest rates of turnover in the United States (Eisnitz, 1997).

> "*If slaughterhouses had glass walls, everyone would be a vegetarian.*"
>
> —Paul McCartney, musician

No one wants to know about the slaughterhouses. They are kept carefully hidden from public view. Few people ever visit these dark places. Many, if not most, countries have no regulation governing the slaughter-houses, while those countries that do have humane slaughter regulations rarely enforce them. In the United States, for example, Congress passed the Humane Slaughter Act in 1958, and this was one of the most popular pieces of legislation in the nation's history; *no sane person* wants animals to suffer needlessly.

The humane slaughter law stipulates that the animal must be knocked unconscious before it is killed. Slaughterhouse workers use a stun gun for this purpose, but unfortunately, the guns frequently fail and break down. The slaughterhouse managers refuse to stop the killing even when the animals cannot be rendered unconscious before the gruesome act. Workers regularly report (and complain) that the cows and pigs are often fully conscious as the metal shackles are fastened around their legs and the machine lifts the terrified animals into the air. Flesh and bones rip and crack. The living, breathing animals move along a conveyor belt upside down, twisting and crying in horrible pain and unimaginable terror, until they reach the place where someone slits their throats. It is an inexcusable tragedy. (Eisnitz, 1997).

> *"In their behavior towards creatures, all men were Nazis. The smugness with which man could do with other species as he pleased exemplified the most extreme racist theories, the principle that might is right."*
>
> —Isaac Bashevis Singer, Nobel prize winner

Even when the stun gun is operating properly, the pain and terror before the mercy of death is extreme. It is a horrendous journey down what slaughterhouse workers call the "kill line." Cows and pigs catch the scent of blood and death the moment they arrive at the slaughterhouse. Cows moan and pigs scream out; they often collapse in helpless terror. Workers use electric prods to force the animals to the place where they are supposed to be knocked unconscious.

A veteran USDA meat inspector from Texas describes what he has seen:

> "Cattle dragged and choked...Knocking 'em four, five, ten times. Every now and then when

> they're stunned they come back to life, and they're up there agonizing. They're supposed to be re-stunned, but sometimes they aren't, and they'll go through the skinning process alive. I've worked in four large [slaughterhouses] and a bunch of small ones. They're all the same. (Eisnitz, 1997).

> "*Before they reach their end, the pigs get a shower, a real one. Water sprays from every angle to wash the farm off them. Then they begin to feel crowded. The pen narrows like a funnel; the drivers behind urge the pigs forward, until one at a time they climb onto the moving ramp... Now they scream... smelling the smells they smell ahead... It was a frightening experience, seeing their fear, seeing so many of them go by, it had to remind me of things no one wants to be reminded of anymore, all mobs, all death marches, all mass murders and executions....*"
>
> —Richard Rhodes, author, *Deadly Feasts*

There is growing scientific evidence that the electric shock renders the animal merely paralyzed but still cognizant of what is happening and fully susceptible to the pain. So, even if the stun gun is used, the mercy of a painless death might not be achieved. (Singer, 2002).

Nor is a humane slaughter granted to the animals killed for kosher meat in accordance with the Jewish dietary laws. This is most unfortunate, for these religious laws sprang from ethical considerations of animal welfare. They were instituted to protect human health and to shield the animals from unnecessary pain, thereby granting them a measure of mercy on the way to the dinner table.

Modern factory farms and the sheer numbers of animals killed combine to make a mockery of the intention of these important laws, and nowadays, some of the most egregious abuses of humane slaughter occur in kosher slaughterhouses (Simon, 2004).

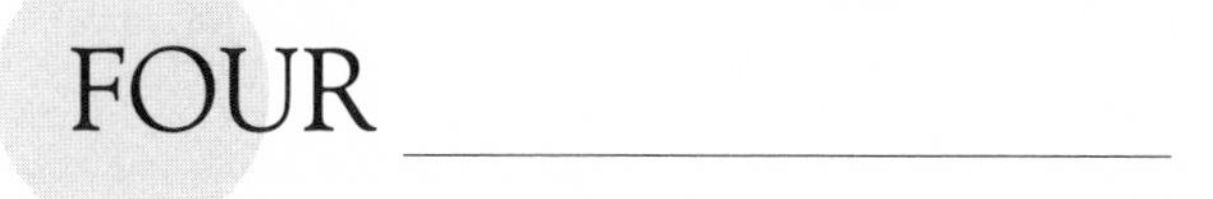

Spiritual and Religious Aspects of Vegetarianism

"A man can live and be healthy without the killing of animals for food: therefore, if he eats meat, he participates in taking an animal's life merely for the sake of his appetite. And to act so is immoral."

—Leo Tolstoy

All religions have strong injunctions against cruelty to animals. The wisest among us have understood the powerful connection between inflicting cruelty and suffering on an animal and the willingness to do the same to people—the thinnest of lines separates the two. The converse is almost always true, and indeed many people have felt or witnessed the depth to which animals connect us to our humanity. Kindness and compassion for animals exercises, and therefore, strengthens our best selves.

> *"The custom of tormenting and killing beasts will, by degrees, harden their hearts even towards men. And, they who delight in the suffering and destruction of inferior creatures, will not be apt to be very compassionate or benign to those of their own kind. Children should from the beginning be brought up in abhorrence of killing or tormenting any living creature."*
>
> —John Locke, philosopher

JUDAISM

The ancient religion of Judaism has strict laws against cruelty to animals. The Jewish kosher laws are both profound and complex, and among the maze of guiding rules and principles, many specifically forbid causing any animal to suffer. The Torah requires that meat and poultry be slaughtered by a process known as *shechita,* a means of causing instantaneous death with no pain to the animal. However, as mentioned before, due to the sheer number of animals killed under kosher rules—*millions*—it is no longer possible to provide a humane slaughter; there is very little true kosher meat. Unfortunately, some of the rabbis in charge of kosher slaughter believe that if they follow the letter of the law, they can ignore its intent.

> *"If animals could talk, would we then dare to kill and eat them? How could we then justify such fratricide?"*
>
> —Voltaire

Many of Judaism's teachings center on caring for human health, treating animals with compassion, ecological conservation, and working toward the alleviation of hunger. Considering the detrimental effects of meat production on each of these concerns, committed Jews will want to move toward vegetarianism. Isaac Singer, the Nobel prize winning novelist, believed that vegetarianism awakened consciousness and purified the soul.

> *"Animals possess a soul, and men must love and feel solidarity with our smaller brethren."*
>
> —Pope John Paul II

CHRISTIANITY

According to the Bible, "And God said, Behold, I have given you every herb-bearing seed, which is upon the face of all the earth, and every tree, in which is the fruit of a tree yielding seed; to you it shall be for meat." (Genesis 1:29)

> *"...They are given into our care, that we cannot just do whatever we want with them. Animals, too, are God's creatures, and even if they do not have the same direct relation to God that man has, they are creatures of his will, creatures we must respect as companions in creation and as important elements in the creation."*
>
> —Pope Benedict XVI

Later in the Bible, God grants Noah's descendants permission to eat meat, but not without grave and unpleasant consequences. Many biblical scholars interpret this to mean that God intended human beings to be vegetarians and that people would do well to follow a plant-based diet. Finally, the Bible predicts that in the messianic age there will be universal vegetarianism, even among normally carnivorous animals. Isaiah 11:7 says, "The cow will feed with the bear, their young will lie down together, and the lion will eat straw like the ox." It should also be noted that many strict cautions against cruelty to animals appear throughout the Bible.

> "*Those who eat flesh are but eating grains and vegetables at second hand; for the animal receives from these things the nutrition that produces growth. The life that was in the grains and the vegetables passes into the eater. We receive it by eating the flesh of the animal. How much better to get it direct by eating the food that God provided for our use!*"
>
> —Ellen White

Additionally, the Bible absolutely forbids the eating of pigs: "Do not eat pigs...They must be considered unclean... (Leviticus 11:1-47; Deuteronomy 14:3-18).

> *"Not to hurt our humble brethren (the animals) is our first duty to them, but to stop there is not enough. We have a higher mission—to be of service to them whenever they require it...If you have men who will exclude any of God's creatures from the shelter of compassion and pity, you will have men who will deal likewise with their fellow men."*
>
> —Saint Francis of Assisi

Many thoughtful Christians believe that vegetarian ethics go hand in hand with Christ's message of love, compassion, and peace, and there is overwhelming evidence that all early church members were vegetarians. Indeed, according to the Essene Gospel of Peace, in a direct translation of early Aramaic texts, Jesus says, "And the flesh of slain beasts in his body will become his own tomb. For I tell you truly, he who kills, kills himself, and whoso eats the flesh of slain beasts, eats the body of death." Several Christian groups encourage vegetarianism, including the Desert Fathers, Trappists, Benedictines, Carthusians, and Seventh Day Adventists.

"*Animals are God's creatures, not human property, nor utilities, nor resources, nor commodities, but precious beings in God's sight...Christians, whose eyes are fixed on the awfulness of crucifixion, are in a special position to understand the awfulness of innocent suffering. The Cross of Christ is God's absolute identification with the weak, the powerless, and the vulnerable, but most of all with unprotected, undefended, innocent suffering.*"

—Rev. Andrew Linzey, professor of theology, Oxford University

ISLAM

The Holy Prophet Mohammed said, "Whoever is kind to the creatures of God is kind to himself," and there is no greater kindness humans can offer animals that the decision to go vegetarian. The Holy Prophet was once asked if kindness to animals was rewarded in the life hereafter, and he replied, "Yes, there is a meritorious reward for kindness to every living creature." The Holy Prophet also said, "It is a great sin for man to imprison those animals which are in his power." Most Imams, those who study the Qu'ran, have concluded that vegetarianism is *halal,* meaning lawful.

"I have no doubt that it is a part of the destiny of the human race in its gradual improvement, to leave off eating of animals as surely as the savage tribes have left off eating each other when they came into contact with the more civilized."

—Henry David Thoreau

HINDUISM

The ancient religion of Hinduism encourages a deep reverence for all living creatures, and a great many Hindus are vegetarians. Like Buddhists and many Christians, Hindus believe animals have souls; they adamantly refuse to consume anything bought at the price of an animal's suffering or death. Gandhi equated the suffering of an animal with that of a person in this way: "The life of a lamb is no less precious than that of a human being. I should be unwilling to take the life of a lamb for the sake of the human body."

"All living beings love their life, desire pleasure, and are averse to pain; they dislike any injury to themselves; everybody is desirous of life, and to every being, his own life is very dear...This is the quintessence of wisdom, not to injure any living being."

—Lord Mahavir, the 24th Tirthankara, or enlightened personage, of the Jain religion

BUDDHISM

The First Precept set down by Buddha prohibits the killing of any living being. "The Blessed One said this to him: For innumerable reasons, Mahamati, the Boddhisattva, whose nature is compassion, is not to eat any meat." Later the Buddha reiterates: "The eating of meat extinguishes the great seed of compassion." He further observes, "All beings tremble before violence. All fear death. All love life."

His Holiness the XIV Dalai Lama has also said, "I do not see any reason why animals should be slaughtered to serve as human diet when there are so many substitutes. After all, man can live without meat."

A story that beautifully illustrates mercy is recorded in this Buddhist sutra:

> A king of heaven was stalemated in a war with a demon, and neither side emerged as winner. As the king of heaven was leading his soldiers back, he saw the nest of a golden-winged bird in a tree by the roadside.
>
> "If the soldiers and chariots pass by here, the eggs in the nest will certainly fall to the ground and be scattered," he thought to himself. So he led his thousand chariots back the same road by which they came. When the demon saw the king of heaven returning, he fled in terror.

Justice for All

The long historical march for social justice is the story of inclusion under the protection of our laws and within an ever-widening circle of our compassion. No longer do we exclude people of different religions, nationalities, people of color, children, or women. Eventually the protective umbrella of our laws will save animals from cruelty. The terrible violence perpetrated against them will finally be at an end, and our kindness will extend to encircle all of earth's creatures. Each person who becomes a vegetarian moves us closer to this ideal.

> "*Vegetarians serve as the criterion by which we know that the pursuit of moral perfection on the part of humanity is genuine and sincere.*"
>
> —Leo Tolstoy

Gandhi stated a universal truth: "The greatness of a nation and its moral progress can be judged by the way its animals are treated. Because animals are voiceless, helpless, and utterly dependent upon humans for their well-being, the measure of any society is how well they are protected from the brutality and suffering imposed by unnatural living conditions."

Arthur Schopenhauer, the great philosopher, points out, "The assumption that animals are without rights, and the illusion that our treatment of them has no moral significance, is a positively outrageous example of Western crudity and barbarity. Universal compassion is the only guarantee of morality." We can all support this international progress by becoming vegetarians.

> *"Whenever I see a meat- and fish-ridden dining table, I know that I am looking upon one of the seeds of war and hatred—a seed that develops into an ugly weed of atrocity... When people ask me, "Is there likely to be a future war?" I answer, "Yes, until the animals are treated as our younger brothers."*
>
> —G. S. Arundale, writer and philosopher

Most people go through life passively observing the world and feeling helpless to effect change and make the world better. Not so vegetarians! We actively participate in shaping the world every day, and this participation is both positive and powerful. Each day becomes an affirmation of the preciousness of life—all of life. In this way, vegetarianism brings greater consciousness to the individual, and this heightened awareness is ultimately far more important than a food choice.

> *"I have from an early age abjured the use of meat, and the time will come when men will look upon the murder of animals as they now look upon the murder of men."*
>
> —Leonardo da Vinci

Fabulous Vegetarian Cookbooks

The American Vegetarian Cookbook from the Fit for Life Kitchen
by Marilyn Diamond

The Complete Italian Vegetarian Cookbook: 350 Essential Recipes for Inspired Everyday Eating
by Jack Bishop, Ann Stratton (Photographer)

The Essential Vegetarian Cookbook
by Rachel Carter

The Everything Vegetarian Cookbook: 300 Healthy Recipes Everyone Will Enjoy *(Everything Series)*
by Jay Weinstein

The Meat-Lover's Vegetarian Cookbook
by Steven Ferry, Tanya Petrovna

The New Farm Vegetarian Cookbook
by Louise Hagler, Dorothy R. Bates

Student's Vegetarian Cookbook, Revised: Quick, Easy, Cheap, and Tasty Vegetarian Recipes
by Carole Raymond

The Starving Students' Vegetarian Cookbook
by Dede Hall

The Teen's Vegetarian Cookbook
by Judy Krizmanic

Vegetarian Times Complete Cookbook
by Vegetarian Times Magazine

The Peaceful Palate
by Jennifer Raymond

Vegetarian 5-Ingredient Gourmet
by Nava Atlas

Quick Vegetarian Pleasures
by Jeanne Lemlin

The Artful Vegan
by Eric Tucker (from Millenium Restaurant in San Francisco)

How it all Vegan!
by Sarah Kramer and Tanya Barnard Arsenal

Cooking with Kurma
by Kurma Dasa

The Voluptuous Vegan
by Myra Kornfeld

Fresh from the Vegetarian Slow Cooker
by Robin Robertson

Vegan Cooking for One
by Leah Leneman

The New Laurel's Kitchen: A Handbook for Vegetarian Cookery and Nutrition
by Laurel Robertson, Carol Flinders, Brian Ruppenthal

Web Sites of Interest

hsus.org—Perhaps the most famous and respected animal rights organization in the U.S. The Humane Society of the United States' web site provides information on all things animal, especially animal welfare issues. You'll find everything from rescuing animals in a disaster and protecting your dog from summer heat to pending wildlife legislation and vegetarian information. This well designed web site is both compelling and informative.

fundforanimals.org—Here is another valuable web site for the animal activist. The Fund for Animals offers information on the world of animal rights, highlighting important ongoing campaigns. Join the ongoing effort to eliminate trap hunting, legislate an end to foie gras, or protect a wildlife area from hunters. They also have an excellent online store.

farmsanctuary.org—Farm Sanctuary's motto: rescue farm animals whenever possible, educate the public about humane farming practices and vegetarian advocacy. Find wonderful heart-warming rescue stories here as well as the case against factory farms and the case for vegetarianism and the humane treatment of all farm animals. Find help here on starting down the vegetarian path. Farm Sanctuary has a good online store as well.

peta.org—People for the Ethical Treatment of Animals is one of the most famous animal rights organizations in the world. PETA never lets a chance for media attention on animal issues slip away, and for this reason PETA is often viewed as somewhat radical. Yet in reality, their determination to stop animal abuse in all its forms is nothing but heroic. This is the place to go for news and information on all aspects of animal rights: factory farms, the abuse of animals in research labs, the use of animals for product testing, fur farms, rescue efforts, all about vegetarianism, and how to turn your concern into action. New vegetarians don't want to miss PETA's free vegetarian starter kit.

petakids.org—PETA for kids! An entertaining, fun and informative web site that introduces kids to the important animal welfare issues of our day.

goveg.com—This is PETA's web site dedicated to all things vegetarian. New vegetarians don't want to miss PETA's free vegetarian starter kit.

earthsave.org—Earthsave International is a worldwide environmental organization founded by John Robbins, author of the excellent book *Diet for a New America*. Earthsave focuses on the environmental destruction caused by meat production and the environmental benefits of vegetarianism. They have interesting and informative articles on vegetarianism and the environment, as well as a great online store. Furthermore, chances are there is a local Earthsave chapter near you for direct involvement in the most important issues of our day.

vegsource.com—This excellent web site offers tons of information on all aspects of vegetarianism and health. It is also a great source of vegan and vegetarian recipes.

furisdead.com—PETA makes the case against fur and for activism against fur.

all-creatures.org/cash—This excellent site is dedicated to the elimination of sport hunting. Find out why—visit.

ethics.acusd.edu/animal.html—Here is an interesting web site that offers an intellectual discussion of the important ethical issues of our day, including animal rights.

animal-rights.com—Another fine source of philosophical subjects, including an excellent question and answer area. There is a powerful and intriguing conversation happening on these pages.

cosmosveganshoppe.com—Find vegan food products, cruelty-free products, and vegan clothing, shoes, and purses. It also maintains an up-to-date animal rights news page.

utilitarian.net/singer—Meet Dr. Peter Singer, professor of bioethics at Princeton University's Center for Human Values, the philosopher who inspired the modern animal rights–vegetarian movement. Some scholars believe Dr. Singer will go down in history as our century's greatest philosopher. Find out why.

api4animals.org—Here is a valuable site for the animal activist. It offers the latest information on new and pending laws to protect animals, both wild and domestic life as well as how people can fight animal abuse in their local communities and in their state legislature.

Web Sites with Vegetarian Recipes

vegweb.com—Find outstanding vegetarian and vegan recipes, as well as vegetarian personals.

vegetarian.allrecipes.com—Find over 800 vegetarian recipes! Don't miss their top ten favorite recipes—excellent. There are also lists of the best vegetarian recipe books and a forum for discussing all things vegetarian.

vegkitchen.com—Nava Atlas, a famous vegetarian chef and vegetarian cookbook author, hosts this excellent web site. Not only does she present hundreds of fabulous vegetarian recipes, but she offers advice on everything from presentation to hosting vegetarian dinner clubs.

ivu.org/recipes—The International Vegetarian Union provides a wealth of information that promotes international vegetarianism. Traveling somewhere in the world where you would like vegetarian dining? This is the place to look. It also offers nearly 2,000 vegetarian recipes from around the world, listed by country. Are you interested in the history of vegetarianism? Were Jesus and the early Christians vegetarians? This is the place for you.

vrg.org—Here is another great source of recipes and information. This site includes a vegetarian game and poll information on vegetarians in the United States.

vegcooking.com—This is PETA's vegetarian web site, packed full of the best vegan recipes, interesting interviews with famous vegetarian chefs, and an informative site for learning how to spread the word.

Suggested Reading

Animal Liberation by Peter Singer

Diet for a New America: How Your Food Choices Affect Your Health, Happiness and the Future of Life on Earth by John Robbins

Dominion: The Power of Man, the Suffering of Animals, and the Call to Mercy by Matthew Scully

Don't Drink Your Milk!: New Frightening Medical Facts About the World's Most Overrated Nutrient by Frank A. Oski

Drawing the Line: Science and the Case for Animal Rights by Steven M. Wise

In Defense of Animals by Peter Singer

Mad Cowboy: Plain Truth from the Cattle Rancher Who Won't Eat Meat by Howard F. Lyman and Glen Merzer

Making Kind Choices: Everyday Ways to Enhance Your Life Through Earth- and Animal-Friendly Living by Ingrid Newkirk

Prisoned Chickens Poisoned Eggs: An Inside Look at the Modern Poultry Industry by Karen Davis

Slaughterhouse by Gail Eisnitz

Skinny Bitch by Kim Barnouin, Rory Freedman

The China Study: The Most Comprehensive Study of Nutrition Ever Conducted and the Startling Implications for Diet, Weight Loss and Long-Term Health by T. Colin Campbell and Thomas M. Campbell II

The Food Revolution: How Your Diet Can Help Save Your Life and Our World by John Robbins

When Elephants Weep: The Emotional Lives of Animals by Jeffrey Moussaieff Masson

References

1. Abelow, B. J., Holford, T. R., & Insogna, K. L. (1992). Cross-cultural association between dietary animal protein and hip fracture: a hypothesis. *Calcified Tissue International, 50*(1), 14-18.

2. Agriculture: Towards 2015/30 technical interim report. (2000). Rome: Food and Agricultural Organization of the UN. Retrieved from http://lnweb18. worldbank.orgESSDardext.nsf/11ByDocName/ AgricultureTowards201530$FILEFAO_2030.pdf# search='agriculture%20towards%20201530%20 Technical%20interim%20report'

3. Anderson, J. W., Johnstone, B. M., & Cook-Newell, M. E. (1995). Meta-analysis of the effects of soy protein intake on serum lipids. *New England Journal of Medicine, 333*(5), 276–282.

4. Appleby, P. N., Thorogood, M., Mann, J. I., & Key, T. J. (1999). The Oxford Vegetarian study: an overview. *American Journal Clinical Nutrition, 70*(Supp), 525S–531S.

5. Barnard, N. D., & Berkow, S. (2005). Blood pressure regulation and vegetarian diets, *Journal of Nutrition Reviews, 1,* 1–8.

6. Barnard, N. D., Nicholson, A., & Howard, J. L. (1995). The medical costs attributable to meat consumption. *Preventative Medicine, 24*(6), 646–655.

7. Barnard, N. D., Scialli, A. R., Hurlock, D., & Bertron, P. (2000). Diet and sex-hormone binding globulin, dysmenorrhea, and premenstrual symptoms. *Obstetrics & Gynecology, 95*(2), 245–250.

8. Bingham, S., & Wilcock, F. (1999). Nutritional aspects of the development of cancer. London: Health Education Authority. Retrieved from http://www.hdaonline.org.uk/ documentsnutritional_devof_ cancer.pdf#search='Nutritional%20 aspects%20of%20the%20development% 20of%20cancer'

9. Bloyd-Peshkin, S. (1991, January/February). "Grazing Our Way to Disaster," *Utne Reader*, 15–16

10. Boyan, S. (2005). How Our Food Choices Can Help Save the Environment. Retrieved Feb 7, 2005 from http://www.vegsource.com/articles/boyan_environment.htm

11. Boyd, N. F., Martin, L. J., Noffel, M., Lockwood, G. A., Trichler, D. L. (1993) A meta-analysis of studies of dietary fat and breast cancer risk. *Journal of Breast Cancer, 68*(3):627–636.

12. Brathwaite, N., Fraser, H. S., Modeste, N., Broome, H., & King, R. (2003). Obesity, diabetes, hypertension, and vegetarians among Seventh-Day Adventists in Barbados: preliminary results, *Ethn Dis. 13*(1), 34–39.

13. Campbell, T. C., & Campbell, T. M. (2006) *The China Study: The Most Comprehensive Study of Nutrition Ever Conducted and the Startling Implications for Diet, Weight Loss and Long-Term Health.* Dallas, TX: BenBella Books.

14. Chang-Claude, J., Frentzel-Beyme, R., & Eilber, U. (1992). Mortality pattern of German Vegetarians after 11 years of follow-up. *Epidemiology, 5,* 395–401.

15. Chang-Claude, J., Hermann, S., Eilber, U., & Steindorf, K. (2005). Lifestyle determinants and mortality in German vegetarians and health-conscious persons: results of a 21-year follow-up. *Cancer Epidemiol Biomarkers Prev., 4,* 963–968.

16. Chao, A., Thun, M. J., Connell, C. J., McCullough, M. L., Jacobs, E. J., Flanders, W. D., Rodriguez, C., Sinha, R., & Calle, E. E. (2005). Meat Consumption and Risk of Colorectal Cancer. *Journal of American Medical Association, 293*(2), 172–182.

17. Cloutier, G. R., & Barr, S. I. (2003). Protein and bone health: literature review and counseling implications. *Can J Diet Prac Rec, 64*(1), 5–11.

18. Cohen, J. H., Kristal, A. R., & Stanford. J. L. (2000). Fruit and vegetable intakes and prostate cancer risk. *J Natl Cancer Inst, 92*(1), 61–68.

19. Cook, M. & Stanley, E. (1998). Reducing Water Pollution from Animal Feeding Operations. Washington, D.C.: US Environmental Protection Agency. Retrieved February 7, 2005 from http://www.epa.gov/ocirpage/hearings/testimony/105_1997_1998/051398.htm

20. Dansinger. M.L., Gleason. J. A., Griffith. J. L., Selker. H. P., & Schaefer. E. J. (2005). Comparison of the Atkins, Ornish, Weight Watchers, and Zone diets for weight loss and heart disease risk reduction: a randomized trial. *Journal of the American Medical Association, 293*(1), 43–53.

21. Deneco-Pellegrini. H., De Stefani. E., Ronco. A., Mendilaharsu, M., & Carzoglio, J. C. (1996). Meat consumption and risk of lung cancer; a case-control study from Uruguay. *Lung Cancer, 14,* 195–205.

22. Diaz-Buxo, J. A. (1998). Optimizing diabetes management. *Adv Perit Dial, 14,* 200–204.

23. Eisnitz, G. A. (1997). *Slaughterhouse.* Amherst: N.Y.: Prometheus Books.

24. EPA's pesticide program: FY 2004 annual report. (2004). Washington, D.C.: US Environmental Protection Agency. Retrieved May 7, 2005 from http://www.epa.gov/oppfead1/annual/2004/04annualrpt.pdf

25. European initiative on harmful algal blooms. (2002, August). Spain: Vigo: Intergovernmental Oceanographic Commission of UNESCO. Retrieved May 7, 2005 from http://ioc.unesco.org/hab/EUROHAB%20HAN%20Issue%202002.PDF#search='European%20initiative%20on%20harmful%20algal%20blooms%20and%20part%20b'

26. Fritschel, H. and Mohan, U. (1999). Are We Ready for a Meat Revolution? 2020 Vision: News and Views. Washington, DC: International Food Policy Research Institute.

27. Giem, P., Beeson, W. L., & Fraser, G. E. (1993). The incidence of dementia and intake of animal products: preliminary findings from the Adventist Health Study. *Neuroepidemiology, 12*(1), 28–36.

28. Giovannucci, E., Rimm, E. B., Colditz, G. A., Stampfer, M. J., Ascherio, A., Chute, C. C., & Willett, W. C. (1993). A prospective study of dietary fat and risk of prostate cancer. *Journal of the National Cancer Institute, 85*(19), 1571–1579.

29. Gorbach, S. L. (2001). Antimicrobial Use in Animal Feed—Time to Stop. *New England Journal of Medicine, 345*(16), 1202–1203.

30. Gussow, J. D. (1994) Ecology and vegetarian considerations: does environmental responsibility demand the elimination of livestock? *American Journal of Clinical Nutrition, 59*(5, Supp), 1110S–1116S.

31. Hall, R. H. (1992). A new threat to public health: organochlorines and food. *Nutrition & Health, 8*(1), 33–43.

32. Halverson, M. (2000). The Price We Pay For Corporate Hogs. Minneapolis, MN: Institute for Agriculture and Trade Policy. Retrieved May 6 2005 from http://www.iatp.org/hogreport/indextoc.html

33. Harada, Y. (1994). Treatment and utilization of animal wastes in Japan. Taipei, Taiwan: Food & Fertilizer Technology Center. Retrieved May 5 2005, from http://www.agnet.org/library/abstract/eb382.html

34. Horrigan, L., Lawrence, R. S., & Walker, P. (2002). How sustainable agriculture can address the environmental and human health harms of industrial agriculture. *Environmental Health Perspectives, 110*(5), 445–456.

35. Howarth, R., Anderson, D., Cloern, J., Elfring, C., Hopkinson, C., Lapointe, B., Malone, T., Marcus, N., McGlathery, K., Sharpley, A., & Walker, D. (2000) Nutrient Pollution of Coastal Rivers, Bays, and Seas. Washington: D.C.: Ecological Society of America. Retrieved May 5 2005 from http://www.esa.org/sbi/sbi_issues/issues_text/issue7.htm

36. Huffman, R. L. & Westerman, P. W. (1995). Estimated Seepage Losses from Established Swine Waste Lagoons in the Lower Coastal Plain in North Carolina, *Transactions of the American Society of Agricultural Engineers, 38*(2), 449–453.

37. Hughes, J., & Norman, R. W. (1992). Diet and calcium stones. *Can Med Assoc J, 146*(2), 137–143.

38. Jenkins, D. J., Kendall, C. W., Marchie, A., Faulkner, D. A., Wong, J. M., de Souza, R., Emam, A., Parker, T. L., Vidgen, E., Lapsley, K. G., Trautwein, E. A., Josse, R. G., Leiter, L. A., & Connelly, P. W. (2003). Effects of dietary portfolio of cholesterol-lowering foods vs lovastatin on serum lipids and C-reactive protein. *JAMA, 290*(4), 502–510.

39. Jenkins, D. J., Kendall, C. W., Marchie, A., Jenkins, A. L., Augustin, L. S., Ludwig, D. S., Barnard, N. D., & Anderson, J. W. (2003) Type 2 Diabetes and the Vegetarian diet. *American Journal of Clinical Nutrition*. 3 (Supp), 610S–616S.

40. Kelleher, C. (2004). *Brain Trust: The Hidden Connection Between Mad Cow and Misdiagnosed Alzheimer's Disease*. New York: Paraview Pocket Books.

41. Kellogg, R. L., et al. (2000). Manure nutrients relative to the capacity of cropland and pastureland to assimilate nutrients: Spatial and temporal trends for the United States. Washington, DC : US Dept. of Agriculture, Natural Resources Conservation Service : Economic Research Service.

42. Key, T. J., Fraser, G. E., Thorogood, M., Appleby, P. N., Beral, V., Reeves, G., Burr, M. L., Chang-Claude, J., Frentzel-Beyme, R., Kuzma, J. W., Mann, J., & McPherson, K. (1998). Mortality in vegetarians and non-vegetarians: a collaborative analysis of 8,300 deaths among 76,000 men and women in five prospective studies. *Public Health Nutrition, 1*(1), 33–41

43. Kjeldsen-Kragh, J., Haugen, M., Borchgrevink, C. F., Laerum, E., Eek, M., Mowinkel, P., Hovi, K., Forre, O. (1991). Controlled trial of fasting and one-year vegetarian diet in rheumatoid arthritis. *Lancet. 338*, 899–902.

44. Kratzer, W., Kachele, V., Mason, R. A., Muche, R., Hay, B., Wiesneth, M., Hill, V., Beckh, K., & Adler, G. (1997). Gallstone prevalence in relation to smoking, alcohol, coffee consumption, and nutrition. The Ulm Gallstone Study. *Scand J Gastroenterol 32*(9), 953–958.

45. Land and Water Resources Research and Development Corporation. [LWRRDC] (2000). Cost of Algal Blooms, Occasional Paper 26/ 99. Canberra Australia: Author. Retrieved May 5, 2005 from http://www.epa.nsw.gov.au/soe/soe2003/chapter5/ chp_5.3.htm#c36.34

46. Livestock Manure Handling on the farm (2002). Washington, D.C.: U. S. Environmental Protection Agency, Retrieved from http:// pasture.ecn.purdue. edu/~epados/farmstead/yards/src/title.htm

47. Livestock on agricultural holdings, Regional Trends 37 (June 2001). United Kingdom: National Statistics Online. Retrieved May 5, 2005, from http://www.statistics.gov.uk/STATBASE/Product.asp?vlnk=5075&More=Y

48. Lyman, H., & Merzer, G. (1998). *Mad Cowboy*. New York: Scribner.

49. Mackay, J., & Mensah, G. (2004). *Atlas of Heart Disease and Stroke.* Switzerland, Geneva: World Health Organization. Retrieved May 7, 2005 from http://www.who.int/cardiovascular_diseases/resources/atlas/en/

50. Malter, M., Schriever, G., & Eilber, U. (1989). Natural killer cells, vitamins, and other blood components of vegetarian and omnivorous men. *Nutr Cancer, 12*(3), 271–278.

51. Mann, J. I., Appleby, P. N., Key, T. J., & Thorogood, M. (1997). Dietary determinants of ischaemic heart disease in health conscious individuals. *Heart, 78 (5)*, 450–455.

52. Marcus, E. (2000). *Vegan: The New Ethics of Eating.* Ithaca, New York: McBooks Press.

53. Marks, R. (2001). Cesspools of shame: How factory farm lagoons and sprayfields threaten environmental and public health. (2001). Washington, D.C.: National Resource Defense Council. Retrieved May 5, 2005 from http://www.nrdc.org/water/pollution/cesspools/cesspools.pdf#search='How%20Factory%20Farm%20Lagoons%20and%20Sprayfields%20Threaten%20Environmental%20and%20Public%20Health,'

54. McDougall, J., Bruce, B., Spiller, G., Westerdahl, J., McDougall, M. (2002). Effects of a low-fat, vegan diet in subjects with rheumatoid arthritis. *Journal of Alternative Medicine 8*(1), 71–75.

55. Melby, C. L., Goldflies, D. G., & Toohey, M. L. (1993). Blood pressure differences in Older Black and White long-term vegetarians and non-vegetarians. *Journal of American College of Nutrition 12*(3), 262–269.

56. Methane: Sources and Emissions (2004). Washington, D.C.: US Environmental Protection Agency. Retrieved May 7, 2005 from http://www.epa.gov/methane/sources.html

57. Meyer, F., Bairati, I., Shadmani, R., Fradet, Y., & Moore, L. (1999). Dietary fat and prostate cancer survival. *Cancer Causes Control, 10*(4), 245–251.

58. Nierenberg, D., & Garcés, L. (2004). Industrial animal agriculture – The next global health crisis. London: World Society for the Protection of animals. Retrieved May 6, 2005 from http://www.wspa.ca/reports/nextglobalcrisis.pdf

59. Pienta, K. J., & Esper, P. S. (1993). Risk factors for prostate cancer. *Ann Intern Medicine, 118*(10), 793–803.

60. Pi-Snyder, F. X. (1991). Health implications of obesity. *American Journal of Clinical Nutrition, 53*(Supp), 1595S–1603S.

61. Prentice, A. M. (1995). Are all calories equal? In: R. C. Cottrell (Ed.) *Weight control: the current perspective.* London: Chapman & Hall.

62. Raloff, J. (2002). Hormones: Here's the Beef: Environmental concerns reemerge over steroids given to livestock. *Science News, 161*(1), 10. Retrieved May 6, 2005 from http://www.findarticles.com/p/articles/mi_m1200/is_1_161/ai_82512511

63. Rifkin, J. (1992). *Beyond Beef: The Rise and Fall of the Cattle Culture*. East Rutherford, NJ: Dutton Books.

64. Risch, H. A., Jain, M., Marret, L. D., & Howe, G. R. (1994). Dietary fat intake and risk of epithelial cancer. *Journal National Cancer Institute 86*(18), 1409–1415.

65. Robbins, J. (1987). *A Diet for a New America.* Novato, CA: New World Library.

66. Sampat, P., & Petersen, J. A. (2000). *Deep Trouble: The Hidden Threat of Groundwater Pollution.* Washington, DC: Worldwatch Institute.

67. Sasaki, S., Zhang, X. H., Kesteloot, H. (1995). Dietary sodium, potassium, saturated fat, alcohol, and stroke mortality. *Stroke 26,*(5), 783–789.

68. Scheierling, S. (1995). *Overcoming Agricultural Pollution of Water: The Challenge of Integrating Agricultural and Environmental Policies in the European Union*. Netlibrary, Inc. Retrieved May 6, 2005 from http://www.bossintl.com/bookstore/index/book/4660.html

69. Schuurman, A. G., van den Brandt, P. A., Dorant, E., & Goldohm, R. A. (1999). Animal products, calcium and protein and prostate cancer risk in the Netherlands Cohort Study. *Br J Cancer 80*(7), 1107–1113.

70. Sellmeyer, D. E., Stone, K. L., Sebastian, A., & Cummings, S. R. (2001). A high ratio of dietary animal to vegetable protein increases the rate of bone loss and the risk of fracture in postmenopausal women. Study of Osteoporotic Fractures Research Group. *American Journal of Clinical Nutrition, 73*(1), 118–122.

71. Simon, S. (2004, December 28). *Los Angeles Times*, p. A.22.

72. Singer, P. (2002) *Animal Liberation*. New York: Harper Collins.

73. Slattery, M. L., Jacobs, D. R. Jr., Hilner, J. E., Caan, B. J., Van Horn, L., Bragg, C., Manolio, T. A., Kushi, L. H., & Liu, K. A. (1991). Meat consumption and its associations with other diet and health factors in young adults: the CARDIA study. *American Journal of Clinical Nutrition, 54*(5), 930–935.

74. Soils, Farming, Forests. (2002). Ottawa, ON: UNA-Canada's "On the Road to Brazil" Series -Issue Paper No.5. Retrieved May 5, 2005, from http://www.unac.org/en/link_learn/monitoring/susdev_archives_land.asp

75. Song, Y., Manson, J. E., Buring, J. E., & Liu, S. (2004). A Prospective Study of Red Meat Consumption and Type Two Diabetes in Middle-aged and Elderly Women. *Diabetes Care 27*(9), 2108–2115.

76. Spinrad, R. (2005, February 16). Testimony to the oversight hearing on NOAA Budget and Priorities for 2006, Washington D.C.: United States House of Representatives. Retrieved May 6, 2005 from http://www.house.gov/transportation/water/02-16-05/spinrad.pdf#search='hearing%20on%20NOAA%20Budget%20and%20Priorities%20for%202006'

77. Thorogood, M., Mann, J., Appleby, P., & McPherson, K. (1994). Risk of death from cancer and ischaemic heart disease in meat and non-meat eaters. *British Medical Journal, 308*, 1667–1670.

78. Thorogood, M., Roe, L., McPherson, K., & Mann, J. (1990). Dietary intake and plasma lipid levels: lessons from a study of the diet of health conscious groups. *British Medical Journal, 300,* 1297–1301.

79. United States Department of Agriculture/Environmental Protection Agency Draft Unified National Strategy for Animal Feeding Operation (1998). Washington, D.C.: National Council of State Legislatures. Retrieved from http://www.ncsl.org/statefed/jtcafosm.htm

80. WHO, Risk Factors: Blood Pressure, World Health Organization, Retrieved May 6, 2005 from http://www.who.int/entity/cardiovascular_diseases/en/cvd_atlas_05_HBP.pdf

81. Zhang, S., Folsom, A. R., Sellers, T. A., Kushi, L. H., & Potter, J. D. (1995). Better breast cancer survival for postmenopausal women who are less overweight and eat less fat. The Iowa Women's Health Study. *Cancer, 76*(2), 275–283.

Index

D

T

About the Authors

Jennifer Horsman and Jaime Flowers are a mother-daughter writing team and enthusiastic vegetarian advocates. Jennifer Horsman is a well-published writer who has written a multitude of romance novels (Avon Books, Zebra Books), several successful screenplays (Warner Bros., Julian Krainin Productions), and weekly book reviews for *Publishers Weekly*. Jaime Flowers is a recent graduate of Chapman University, where she majored in film and screenwriting.

Please visit
PleaseDontEatTheAnimals.com
&
QuillDriverBooks.com